No More Periods?

Also by Susan Rako, M.D.

THE HORMONE OF DESIRE:
THE TRUTH ABOUT TESTOSTERONE,
SEXUALITY, AND MENOPAUSE

No More Periods?

The Risks of Menstrual Suppression
and Other Cutting-Edge Issues About
Hormones and Women's Health

Susan Rako, M.D.

Harmony Books / New York

The information in this book is educational in nature and is not intended to substitute for or to supersede individual, responsible medical consultation.

Published by Harmony Books, New York, New York.
Member of the Crown Publishing Group, a division of Random House, Inc.
www.randomhouse.com

Harmony Books is a registered trademark and the Harmony Books colophon is a trademark of Random House, Inc.

Printed in the United States of America

Design by Jennifer Ann Daddio

Library of Congress Cataloging-in-Publication Data
Rako, Susan.
No more periods? : the risks of menstrual suppression and other cutting-edge issues about hormones and women's health / Susan Rako.
Includes index.
1. Menstruation—Prevention—Health aspects.   2. Contraceptive drugs—Health aspects.   3. Women—Health and hygiene.
I. Title.
QP263.R35   2003
618.1'72—dc21   2002155720

ISBN 1-4000-4503-7

10 9 8 7 6 5 4 3 2 1

First Edition

To my grandparents,
with gratitude
for their courage and foresight in leaving
their homelands and crossing the ocean
to make a life in America
for themselves and their posterity.

Acknowledgments

I wish to thank my extraordinary daughter (who is, as well, an extraordinary mother and attorney), Ms. Jennifer S. Rako, for her loving and generous gift of a critical review of the completed manuscript. Dearest Jenni, you nourished my spirit when I needed it most. No author could have a more exquisitely discerning, respectful, balanced, and intelligent reader.

I wish to thank Ms. Jane Broderick for her diligent help shoulder to shoulder in the stacks and at the copy machines at Countway, for her painstaking work with the References section, and for her sense of humor always.

I appreciate my inspired and inspiring editor, Ms. Shaye Areheart, for knowing the value of this book from the first. We are blessed with the gift of profound mutual respect.

I wish to thank my friend Ms. Jeanne Mayell, who saw me through the anguishing aspects of this difficult project with brilliance and love, and without whose acute understanding the book would not be what it is.

I wish to acknowledge Ms. Dara Arons for her generosity, creative intelligence, integrity, responsibility, and grace in soliciting and conducting interviews with physicians and women. She will be a doctor women can trust.

My gratitude to Ms. Lisa Resnek for directing me to Mary Wollstonecraft's treatise on the rights of women.

I wish to thank the physicians and women who contributed their knowledge, wisdom, hard-won experiences, and time.

I wish to acknowledge Ms. Deborah Rose, Drs. Elissa and Daniel Arons, Ms. Linda Land, Dr. Jay Land, Ms. Gregoria Scheier, Dr. Allen Scheier, Dr. Manya Arond-Thomas, Mr. John Taylor, Ms. Colette Taylor, Mr. Peter Taylor, Ms. Marie Harburger, Dr. Irwin Avery, my outstanding son-in-law, Mr. Thomas Bernardo, and other beloveds who dependably travel the path with me with patience, love, and pleasure.

My thanks to Dr. Jonathan Moreno, Dr. Paul Applebaum, Dr. Thomas Gutheil, Dr. George Kornitzer, Ms. Lisa Hutchins, Ms. Ali Kedge, Ms. Alison Motluk, and Ms. Harriet Jump for their willing and helpful responses to queries.

And I thank Ms. Ezila Do Canto for her abundant loving help, and Mr. Michael Meltzer and Mr. Andrew Meltzer for their assistance in loading and unloading the printer, books, and papers, and much else in to and out of my car at critical junctures.

Contents

Without knowledge there
can be no morality!

MARY WOLLSTONECRAFT

A Vindication of the Rights of Woman (1792)

A Letter to Dr. Rako on Menstrual Suppression

I have grave concerns about the wisdom of menstrual suppression, which could chemically suppress the feminine cycle of sex-hormone secretion—turning it into the malelike, flatter, less cyclically evolved sex-hormone pattern. All sex hormones affect physiological systems, including cardiovascular health, bone metabolism, cognitive function, sexual response, and sexual attractiveness. The fertile menstrual cycle serves more than just the next generation. A fertile pattern of hormonal secretion promotes general health and well-being. This coordinated pattern is well illustrated in a graceful sequence of fluctuating ebbs and flows of blood-borne hormones secreted from the ovary: the estrogens, progesterone, and testosterone. And with this rhythmic cyclic alteration in the sex hormones come consequent alterations in psychodynamic events, such as dreaming, energy, and cognition.

Physicians who care for women as patients should under-stand the interplay between sex hormones and their well-being. The peer-reviewed literature, whether focused on metabolic bone diseases, cardiovascular health, atherosclerotic processes, immunology, sexual-response cycles, or studies of cognition, continues to reveal complex associations among physiology, behavior, and sex hormones. Cyclic secretion of estrogen, progesterone, testosterone, androstenedione, and DHEA(S) play significant roles in maintaining the cascade of physiological events that promote healthy bone metabolism, sexual interest and response, and cardiovascular function, as well as adequate sleep and energy cycles. Ovarian hormones influence diverse neuroendocrine pathways: Beta endorphins, melatonin, oxytocin, growth hormone, prostaglandins, and the adrenal androgens (including DHEA[S]) are all increasingly being identified as intimately dependent upon the cyclic secre-tions of ovarian hormones. Excessively high or low levels of the hormones are associated with many diseases.

Estrogen has been shown to play a structural role in the central nervous system, interacting with progesterone to help maintain both nerves and myelinization. And now it seems that the cyclic progesterone of a fertile menstrual cycle is responsi-ble for triggering other hormone secretions such as oxytocin, which, in turn, enhances sexual sensation of uterine and breast tissue by enhancing contractility. Fertile cycles promote the excretion of sex-attractant pheromones. Oral contraceptives that are monophasic suppress (flatten) the cyclic rise and fall of sex hormones and have negative effects on sexual interest (libido), in contrast to the triphasics, which yield better sexual response in women.

Bones represent another concern. The life history of a healthy woman's bone shows the period of rapid pubescent growth of long bones to conclude when the end plates close shortly after puberty. Thereafter, provided her calcium intake exceeds the obligatory daily calcium excretion (estimated at about 600 mgs per day), and her health and habits are good, with regular monthly ovulatory menstrual cycles, her bones continue to accrete mineral by thickening instead of lengthening through her midthirties. The thicker the bone she is able to build, the less vulnerable to fracture she will be during her menopausal years.

The regulation of bone remodeling involves a continual cycling of bone resorption and bone formation and is under the control of hormones and other factors that include mechanical stress, inorganic phosphate levels, and plasma calcium levels. The rate of bone formation diminishes at the same time of life that the fertile rhythm of the menstrual cycle moves into the aging pattern of the perimenopausal transition years, usually around age forty. Once the dynamic processes of bone resorption and bone formation are no longer closely linked (termed uncoupled bone remodeling), bone loss occurs.

Experts suggest that bone remodeling is closely coupled to the ovarian cycle of the fertile years, and that a high (29 percent) rate of ovulatory disturbance, generally unappreciated by either the woman or her physician, occurs in twenty- to forty-five-year-old healthy women. The consequence of these hidden ovulatory disturbances is a dramatically declining spinal bone density in young women. Young women develop old women's bones. Progesterone in cyclic opposition to estrogen is not yet universally appreciated for its essential role in bone metabolism. Hence it is an informed concern that menstrual suppression will have long-term negative effects on bone remodeling.

Traditional medical practices have long focused upon disease treatment, which necessarily pays insufficient respect to the importance of learning how the exquisite female cycle, so rich and complex, may contribute to the increased life span women enjoy in comparison with their male counterparts.

The natural fertility cycle is a great gift of nature. Until each of the above-captioned physiologic systems has been carefully tested for adverse effects of "menstrual suppression," I would remind all of us of the wisdom of the Hippocratic Oath: ABOVE ALL, DO NO HARM. For now, I would caution my daughters and granddaughters: Revel in the cycles of your youth. They are the key to your health, your sex-attractant pheromones, your longevity, your very femininity.

Winnifred B. Cutler, Ph.D.,
President and Founder,
The Athena Institute for Women's Wellness
Chester Springs, Pennsylvania
www.athenainstitute.com

No More Periods?

Foreword

The *New Yorker* of March 13, 2000, has a yellow cover with an amusing cartoon of the evolution of man from monkey to pot-bellied, visor-capped human male. It also features "John Rock's Error," an article by Malcolm Gladwell with the focus "What the co-inventor of the Pill didn't know: menstruation can endanger women's health"—a radical assertion that demands broad and thorough evaluation. Gladwell is the author of the then-recently-published *The Tipping Point* (a phrase taken from the world of epidemiology—the name given to that moment in an epidemic when a virus reaches critical mass). Gladwell's book develops the concept that "ideas and products and messages and behaviors spread just like viruses do."

The disturbing reality is that the unexamined idea of the "benefits" of menstrual suppression *is* making its way through our society like a disease. Doctors have been prescribing existing oral contraceptive pills "off-label" (for uses other than those approved by the Food and Drug Administration), and pharmaceutical companies have in the pipeline drugs designed for menstrual suppression. One form of contraception has been doing away with periods for a decade and thinning adolescents' and *young* women's bones in the process. Methods of menstrual suppression already in use put women at increased risk for osteoporosis, infertility, heart attacks, strokes, and cancer. Beyond these dangers to women's health, hormonal interruption of the menstrual cycle affects female-male partner choice, is intimately linked with factors that determine immune mechanisms, and can ultimately even detrimentally affect the human species.

In addition to the popular ignorance about the serious risks of suppressing the menstrual cycle is the popular ignorance of the particular health *benefits* that accrue to women as a result of normal hormonal fluctuations and of the monthly bleed. In addition to the fact that women's reproductive hormones play a part in the normal functioning of every organ system in the body are two little-known specific advantages (and it is likely that there are other physiological advantages yet to be discovered) of women's natural hormonal rhythms:

- Effective reduction in blood pressure during half of the normal menstrual cycle, and
- Reduction of stored iron, with concomitant reduced risks for heart attacks and strokes.

Dr. Jerome Sullivan's "iron hypothesis" (which will be presented in full in Chapter Three) has, for twenty years, been evolving through Schopenhauer's *Stages of Truth:*

All truths pass through three stages.
  First, they are ridiculed;
  Second, they are violently opposed;
  Third, they are accepted as being self-evident.

I know the matter well. Fifteen years ago I began the tough and, in its early years, lonely trek researching and teaching about the fundamental role of testosterone in female physiology. This unexpected path had opened to me when I was challenged by my own experience of menopause:

*When I was forty-seven, still having menstrual periods—albeit irregularly—and several years **before** the eventuation of my menopause, I could not make sense of the significant loss in general vital energy, thinning and loss of pubic hair, and loss of sexual energy I experienced. To say that I was lacking a feeling of well-being would be an understatement.*

. . . I was not inclined to settle for the temporizing, patronizing, dismissive, and irresponsibly uninformed treatment I received from the gynecologists and endocrinologists I consulted.

In a search to learn what I could find about loss of sexual and vital energy at menopause, I became very familiar with the stacks of Harvard's Countway Medical Library and of several other libraries.

The data was there

**But it didn't say estrogen was what I needed.
It said testosterone.**

> —*The Hormone of Desire:*
> *The Truth About Testosterone,*
> *Sexuality, and Menopause*

Only a few years ago, many physicians considered the prospect of testosterone supplementation for women suffering symptoms of testosterone deficiency to be "ridiculous." That testosterone is essential for women's health and quality of life (manifested in energy, mood, and sexual sensitivity and response) has made it to "self-evident" (in Schopenhauer's hierarchy) to a large and growing sector of women and health-care professionals is, for me, an immeasurably important and rewarding evolution. I'm afraid that it will take longer for the cardioprotective benefits as well as the full range of health-maintenance functions of normal levels of testosterone (both in women and in men) to be acknowledged as self-evident. I am confident that that time will come.

It had never been my dream to become an authority in the field of women's hormonal health. When I had spent more than a decade significantly committed to this work, I was ready to turn my attention away from reproductive physiology and back to a book of essays and stories from my life. That's when the idea of the "benefits" of menstrual suppression began making its way through our society very much like a disease does. From the vantage (ad- and dis-) of knowing what I know about hormones and women's physiology, I felt compelled to explore the matter fully and to put into perspective the medical implications and the risks to women of the sort of tampering with the natural order that is in the works. Ah, well. The essays and stories are on hold once again. . . .

What Malcolm Gladwell did not address, what the media has not conveyed, what the public has not heard, what too few health professionals know, and what every woman and her doctor MUST know about the hazards of menstrual suppression deserves a voice.

I am determined that it will have one.

Chapter 1

No More Periods?

● ● ● ● ●

THE WASHINGTON POST
SEPTEMBER 7, 2000

A Pill to Uncramp Women's Style
Libby Copeland, Staff Writer

I think we have to disabuse health professionals and women of the idea that monthly menstruation is natural, normal and healthy.

Dr. David Grimes
University of North Carolina
Professor of Gynecology

We're into the era of medicine making life more convenient.

Dr. Charlotte Ellertson

The Lancet

March 11, 2000

Nuisance or natural and healthy: should monthly menstruation be optional for women?

Continuous use of ordinary oral contraceptives safely lets women control . . . whether and when they choose to bleed.

When such a safe, simple, and inexpensive treatment is already so widely available, women should not have to be driven loony by their lunar cycles if they prefer not to bleed each month.

> Charlotte Ellertson, Ph.D.
> Population Council, Latin
> America and the Caribbean
> *"thanks to Elsimar Coutinho for*
> *ideas and suggestions"*

Chicago *Daily Herald*

December 11, 2000

No More Period. Period.
Lorilyn Rackl, *Daily Herald* Health Writer

Unless you're trying to get pregnant, there's no physiological reason to have a monthly period.

The drum beat for fewer periods definitely is getting louder, leaving some experts to predict the feminine hygiene aisles at Wal-Mart will one day be a lot less crowded.

I know the tampon and pad people don't want to hear this. I routinely put women on birth control pills and have

*them not take their last week's pills to suppress their peri-
ods. A lot of them love it.*

> Dr. Teresa Ann Hoffman
> Gynecologist
> Mercy Medical Center
> Baltimore

*I have this box of tampons in my cupboard and I told my
sister the other day, "God, I gotta throw these out, because
they're so old they'd probably be dangerous."*

*The longer you go without a period, the more you real-
ize you didn't need it. There's a certain freedom to not having to plan Kotex in your luggage.*

> Leslie Miller, M.D.
> Assistant Professor
> Obstetrics/Gynecology
> University of Washington

From the "Health Science" section of my hometown news-
paper—full page:

THE BOSTON GLOBE
AUGUST 22, 2000, MEGAN SCOTT, GLOBE CORRESPONDENT

NO chocolate cravings
No PMS or bloating
No fatigue or moodiness
What if having your period
was a choice?

It's up to you

This article goes on to quote Dr. Freedolph Anderson, director of clinical research at the Institute for Reproductive Medicine of Eastern Virginia Medical School:

There's really no good medical reason for menstruation.

THE WALL STREET JOURNAL
JUNE 25, 2002

Doctors Push New Efforts to Eliminate Women's Periods
Tara Parker-Pope, in "Health Journal"

If we're not offering it [period suppression] routinely to women, they don't know this is an option. They don't know how healthy it can be for them.

> Anita Nelson, M.D.
> Professor of Obstetrics and
> Gynecology
> University of California at Los
> Angeles

The *Boston Globe* article describes Dr. Anderson as "one of the leaders of the anti-period movement, overseeing a nationwide test of a form of birth-control pill that would reduce the number of periods a woman has each year from 13 to 4."

"Anti-period movement?"

For years I have been sickened by the irresponsibility of media-coined "official" categories. One particular bizarre or obscene event can be neutralized of its impact when it is referred to as just another example of a created "category." Naming is a form of tacit acceptance of the unacceptable.

"Car-jacking." "Drive-by shooting." "Ethnic cleansing."

By comparison, "anti-period movement" sounds, but is not, innocuous. Disturbing, too, for women's natural lunar cycle to be considered an appropriate subject for social-economic-political positioning. When first I read the words, I thought, What's next—an "anti–high tide/low tide movement? Not much is safe from "improvement." Since my research and teaching about the function of testosterone in women's physiology, and following the publication of my book *The Hormone of Desire: The Truth About Testosterone, Sexuality, and Menopause,* I have had several reorienting experiences.

One, in particular, stands out. June 1998. Washington, D.C. I am preparing to speak at the Congress on Women's Health. In the lobby, I am introduced to a physician who consults to the Food and Drug Administration. The first words he says to me: "I hear that we are on different sides of the coin." He knows that I see the need for FDA-approved, properly dosed pharmaceutical preparations of testosterone for women suffering symptoms of testosterone deficiency—and his comment implies that he holds some opposing position. "I am concerned with *the whole coin,*" I tell him levelly. And I mean it.

Interesting metaphor, though: *coin.* I am a realist. Our democratic and capitalist society, which I honor and choose over any other on earth, benefits from pharmaceutical companies' investment in research and development of new drugs. However, the fact that drug companies fund a significant percentage of research projects (and the scientific papers that they generate) creates a potential for bias and manipulation of publications in medical journals.

This problem of potential bias in scientific publications has become of such substantial concern that editors-in-chief of *thirteen* of the most prominent medical journals authored, in one voice, an extraordinary and comprehensive editorial published in the autumn of 2001 in the *Journal of the American Medical Association,* the *Lancet,* the *British Medical Journal, Obstetrics and Gynecology,* and half a dozen others. Their notable effort addressed the wide range of potential conflict of interest—political, personal, economic, and other on the part of contributing authors, "peer reviewers" (who have the power to accept or reject a paper for publication), and of editors themselves. The editorial said:

> *If a study is funded by an agency with a proprietary or financial interest in the outcome, editors may ask authors to sign a statement such as, "I had full access to all of the data in this study and I take complete responsibility for the integrity of the data and the accuracy of the data analysis." Editors should be encouraged to review copies of the protocol and/or contracts associated with project-specific studies before accepting such studies for publication. Editors may choose not to consider an article if a sponsor has asserted control over the authors' right to publish.*

These reasonable suggestions are not yet universal rules. The arena of scientific publications today has a way to go toward dependable integrity. When we read or hear in the media a report of the findings of some recent study, it might be helpful if we were told who sponsored the research.

Obviously, scientists and clinicians work and publish papers on subjects of special interest to them. In promoting a particular theory or pharmaceutical approach, researchers sometimes focus on the drawbacks of competing theories or pharmaceuticals. Sometimes that's a good thing. When conducted and reported with integrity, studies motivated by an intention to expose the shortcomings and risks of competing theories and pharmaceuticals can contribute important information to understanding the whole picture.

While the knowledge and ethical standards of vigilant editors of scientific journals can help to protect that arena from distorting bias, the media's communication of news about medical-scientific subjects presents a different challenge. News articles regularly report breaking developments in medical science. However, at times a particular feature is mistaken in emphasis or significantly incomplete. Part of the job of journalists (and their editors) is to draw our attention, of course. And news writers—even the best ones—cannot be authorities on every one of the subjects they report. The dramatic headlines and the slant of news stories featuring "no more periods" is a solid example of this limitation.

My first contact with "the anti-period movement" was the Gladwell article mentioned in the Foreword, whose subtitle, "Menstruation Can Be Dangerous to a Woman's Health," is arresting and, with an emphasis on the qualifying verb, technically accurate. It certainly got my attention. The implication of this message is that women can be better off NOT menstruating. Women can also be worse off. Menstrual suppression can be dangerous to a woman's health.

The consequences of manipulating a woman's natural, complex hormonal chemistry by dosing her more or less nonstop with birth control pills—a method of menstrual suppression that is in active development—concerns me greatly. While I was reading the *New Yorker* piece, I had a visceral response: nausea and fear. My female nature shouted an intuitive "NO" as my brain began to spin with what I knew to be some of the implications for our intricate physiological chemistry. In some "thought-form shorthand" version, this is what raced through my mind (it is technical language that probably won't mean

much without the translation that will come later, but may give
a flavor of what got me going on this subject):

> *How can anyone believe that disrupting the menstrual cycle*
> *is innocuous? Constant estrogen stimulation decreases*
> *ACTH and increases binding proteins, leading to lowered*
> *DHEAS levels and lowered available testosterone levels.*
> *Disrupting the normal menstrual cycle eliminates a natural*
> *mechanism that lowers blood pressure. These changes are*
> *bad for our immune system and our response to stress,*
> *increase our risk of heart attacks and strokes, and decrease*
> *our sexual desire, sensitivity, and pleasure.*
>
> *Manipulating women's natural hormonal chemistry*
> *messes with the basis of sexual attraction and partner*
> *choice between women and men, with consequences that are*
> *linked to and can even detrimentally affect the genetic*
> *inheritance of immune mechanisms for our human species.*
>
> *Motivating women to use oral contraceptives for the*
> *purpose of menstrual suppression puts increased numbers of*
> *sexually active women—including very young women—at*
> *risk for potentially lethal sexually transmitted diseases. It's*
> *not just the AIDS virus that's threatening us. Women are*
> *dying from cancer of the cervix caused by high-risk strains*
> *of the Humanpapilloma Virus (HPV).*

The title of a book by Brazilian gynecologist Dr. Elsimar
Coutinho, *Is Menstruation Obsolete?,* hones in on *menstrual
bleeding*—as though that part of the female hormonal cycle can
be isolated from the whole and simply done away with. Of
course it cannot. "No more periods" is where the folks on the
bandwagon of "the anti-period movement" want the spotlight.
What they are actually proposing (and presenting as though it

were an innocuous manipulation) is NO MORE MEN-
STRUAL CYCLE.

What is at issue here is not only the monthly bleed, but the
whole of the natural female reproductive cycle. The intricate
interplay of hormones that rise and fall in a monthly pattern
have remarkable effects on every organ system in the body and
are at the foundation of natural and sexual selection in the
human species.

Imagine the television ads for one of the new pharmaceuticals: images of carefree and happy women active in sports
intercut with scenes of romance. Voice-over: "No more periods." And then, very small print at the bottom of the screen
and very, very fast voice-over:

> *This medication has been shown to increase the risk of
> blood clots, heart attacks, and strokes, to interfere with sex-
> ual desire and pleasure, to increase the user's risk of cancer
> of the cervix, to expose the user to infection with sexually
> transmitted diseases, to alter the chemistry of male-female
> attraction. . . .*

We need more than a voice-over to understand the hazards
of menstrual suppression. We need a careful, knowledgeable,
balanced, responsible, unhurried voice.

Chapter 2

The Blessings of the Curse

"Growing Up and Liking It" was, back in "the olden days" of my childhood—the 1940s and '50s—a pamphlet produced by one of the sanitary napkin companies. When I was about eleven, my mother gave me the booklet, together with a pink elastic sanitary belt that had extensions with small *W*-shaped attachers for the gauze ends of sanitary napkins. I remember those pages, their matter-of-fact tone, the illustrations of the growing-up-girls, the diagrams of the ovaries and the uterus, and the explanation that went something like this:

> *When a girl grows up and becomes a young woman, each month her ovaries mature an egg, and her womb prepares a lining bed for the egg to plant. If the egg does not become fertilized, the lining of the womb sheds. This shedding is called a menstrual period.*

Aha! So that's what those mysterious boxes neatly wrapped in unmarked brown paper and stacked in a corner of my father's grocery store were, and what they were really for.

Neither the first nor the last of the girls in my seventh-grade class, I began menstruating at twelve and a half. I remember the time as an unusual "private/public" event in my large extended family. My much older cousin Dorothy and her husband, Jimmy, came by for a visit, and I didn't tell them—but my mother must have—because there was a subtle difference in the air. I was a little bit embarrassed, and a little bit proud.

I remember, too, the paraphernalia involved in dressing up for the ballroom dancing class on Saturday nights at Temple Emanuel. Once a month I had another belt to wear underneath the garter belt with its dangling gizmos that held up my nylons. I didn't have much of a belly in those days, but, like my friends, if I wore a "straight skirt," I wore a panty girdle.

And in eighth-grade Latin class, one of the taller boys who had pimples (I know now that this meant his testosterone was surging) drew the girls' attention in an original way. Early in the year, our Latin teacher taught us the Lord's Prayer, by rote, in Latin. We recited it nearly every day. By today's standards, that would be pretty strange. No, I guess it would be impossible. But in public school, in Worcester, Massachusetts, in 1952, each morning we said the Lord's Prayer in English and saluted the flag, and some teachers read a daily verse from the Bible that sat on their desks next to the dictionary. Anyway, in eighth grade, I learned the Lord's Prayer in Latin. The beginning sounded something like: Pahter Noster kwee et in chayliss Ko-tid-ee-anum novum too-um . . .

As soon as we got to the "Ko-tid-ee-anum," this pimply kid used to whisper to the girls, pretty loud, "Kotex, Ko-tex" . . . and the other boys would giggle. He did get my attention. Fifty years ago, and I remember this, but I don't remember his name.

At school, too, there was something hush-hush about a girl's not jumping into the swimming pool during gym. *She's having her period.* I remember reading Anne Frank's *Diary of a Young Girl,* where she referred to her menstrual period as her "sweet secret." I much preferred these earnest and tender words to the occasionally heard and, I thought, ugly term "the curse"— which was, both in my personal experience and from what I knew of my girlfriends' experiences, not fitting. Crude and confusing, actually. I knew that menstruation was what we could see of a woman's role in the big picture of having babies, and I simply couldn't consider this aspect of women's nature to be a curse.

When the chapter title "The Blessings of the Curse" occurred to me, I thought it had a nice ironic ring to it. I am prepared for the possibility that, like *The Hormone of Desire,* it will be used as a headline, or subtitle, or catchy phrase for some feature articles that make mention neither of the book nor its author. I have never found solace in the idea that "imitation is the sincerest form of flattery." I wonder who ever thought about pairing "sincerity" with "flattery"? Who wants flattery, anyway? Simple and fair acknowledgment would be fine.

Of course I learned early on that life isn't simple and often isn't fair. While I was personally blessed with healthy reproductive physiology, I was not immune to the political disadvantage of being female. When, in 1961, as a young married college graduate I applied to medical school, an admissions interviewer at Harvard was surprisingly open with me about the unwritten policy of the times.

You qualify for admission. But I'll be honest with you—you won't be admitted. We are just not admitting married women.

We don't want to take the risk that they might get pregnant and drop out.

"Wait-listed" at Harvard (I would have had to wait a few years for their policy manifestly to change), I was relieved, to be sure, when the first of four acceptance letters arrived from other medical schools.

Harvard's concern turned out to be half-correct. I did get pregnant and have a baby. But I did not drop out of medical school. Of the one hundred students in my first-year class at Albert Einstein College of Medicine, seven were women. By the time we graduated, five of us were married and had had babies. One woman had even managed to have two. For better and for worse, none of us dropped out. Harvard's admissions policy hadn't given sufficient weight to the determination of women who chose to become doctors in those days. Oh—come to think of it—one woman did quit, though. She was a nun.

In my fourth year of medical school, I was accepted for a six-month elective period rotating through various teaching hospitals in Harvard's department of psychiatry, and in 1967, I was the one woman in a group of twenty-five first-year residents accepted to Massachusetts Mental Health Center, at the time Harvard's elite psychiatric training program. It was very fine. There I found a mentor in the extraordinary teacher Dr. Elvin Semrad, who understood life and living better than anyone else I have known. Dr. Semrad's wisdom is excerpted in sutras, epigrams, and comments that a colleague and I collected and published after his death in 1976; more than twenty years later, it is still in print.

When I knew him, Dr. Semrad was in his sixties, looked older, and was . . . well . . . fat. He was also rather a courtly man.

Altogether respectful and appropriate, and actually formal in his way of relating, he often had a twinkle in his eye that made me feel glad I was a woman. I heard that he was still buying stockings with seams up the back for his equally heavyset wife, Rita, in the 1970s, when that style of hosiery had been out of vogue for at least twenty years. I smile to think of it.

From the time I was a girl, it had seemed to me that to be a woman was special in positive ways. During the years of my childhood, the 1940s, men (military *and* civilian) wore hats, tipped them for a lady, stood when a woman entered a room, and gave her a seat on the bus—even if she wasn't nine months pregnant. I felt that those customs reflected, on a deeper level, a respect for the mysteries of the female—of which having one's period was a fundamental manifestation.

When I was a freshman in college and in the intimacy of dorm living at Wellesley, I got to know that suffering could be a miserable accompaniment to menstruation for some girls. A junior girl who lived up the hall had horrible pain with her period each month. Her normally pale white skin took on a greenish hue, and she curled up in bed with a hot water bottle trying to ease terrible cramps. While the rest of us took our periods in stride, Molly repeatedly endured what could fairly be described as an accursed ordeal.

With what I know today about reproductive physiology, and remembering the specifics of how she looked and felt, I can speculate that Molly's body was producing high levels of prostaglandins, which today's anti-prostaglandins (like ibuprofen) might have helped. Or maybe she had endometriosis, a miserable condition in which tissue normally found only in the lining of the uterus has planted itself on other organs in the abdomen, where it bleeds and causes pain during menstruation.

Molly was laid low every month to the point that, had menstrual suppression been an option for her, it could well have been worth the risks. I certainly believe that, if a girl or woman suffers from endometriosis or from an illness (such as some conditions of menstrual migraine headaches and some forms of epilepsy) that is improved by intervention for hormonal stability, a carefully selected method of menstrual suppression is worth trying. In those instances, the benefits may well be worth the risks.

The majority of us blessed with normally functioning bodies take our rhythms so much for granted that we may not fully appreciate the aspects of sensuality, sexuality, energy, and creativity that constitute our nature. As we grow older, it's not uncommon to hear that *youth is wasted on the young*. There's a little bitterness in those words—or maybe just wistfulness. And it is, actually, a sort of silly phrase, since a hallmark of youth is a sense of endless possibilities. To appreciate what we have while we have it requires us both to live in the present moment and to accept the end of each moment dying into the next— wisdom not commonly available before our lives have been tempered by loss and grief of some degree. Youthful health is granted to most of us, and we cannot know what it is *not* to have the clear energy of youth until it begins to wane.

For myself, at sixty-two, having enjoyed a fertile lifetime of untroubled female physiology, borne a child, found my way through and learned from a challenging perimenopause, and now eleven years past menopause and supplementing estrogen and testosterone modestly, I feel fine—for sixty-two. Still, I remember the crystal-clear energy of my reproductive years, the "nesting instinct" that impelled me to clean house near the end of an occasional month's cycle, the surge of sexual desire I pretty regularly experienced for the couple of days before a monthly bleed, my need for quiet and rest, and a feeling of natural vulnerability during menstrual days.

In the spring of one year when I was in my late forties, when I was having very irregular periods and not likely ovulating, I had the gift of one month that felt, in my body in all its aspects, like the days of my younger womanhood. I figure that I must have ovulated that month, and I enjoyed, for the first time in several years, the experience of one "regular" menstrual cycle. I felt truly wonderful.

Around that time, as part of the research for *The Hormone of Desire,* I was interviewing gynecologists. One delightful, experienced, and very smart "old time doc" from Worcester, Dr. Saul Lerner, told me that, over decades of practice, he had observed that "women's bodies perk up in the spring." Each subsequent year, I looked forward to the spring, but, alas, my aging woman's body did not perk up in just that way again.

There is a time to sow and a time to reap. There is a time for youth and a time for age. The poetry of Ecclesiastes has an apt rhythm. During our female reproductive years, there is a time for each phase of an incredibly intricate cycle—the hormonal cycle that affects every organ system in our bodies. To tamper with that "time," to interrupt our natural rhythms, has physiological costs—some measurable and known (or available to be known, if we take the trouble to look) and others that can and will be known only with the passage of time. Perhaps when it is too late.

In 1959, biologists first described their observation that animals have glands that excrete substances that influence the social and sexual behavior of other animals that sniff them. They called these substances pheromones. Pheromones differ from hormones in the following way: Hormones are substances that are secreted by glands of an animal or person into the bloodstream of that animal or person and produce effects on other tissues of that same animal or person's body; pheromones are substances that are produced by glands (of an animal or person) that excrete the substances onto the skin and into the air, where they produce effects on *another* animal or person. A newborn baby, for example, can recognize its mother through the pheromones her body produces.

In 1971, a decade after my undergraduate years at Wellesley, a fellow Wellesley alumna, Martha McClintock, published a paper in the journal *Nature* that described her observation that the young women who lived together in her dormitory and shared bathroom facilities appeared to synchronize their menstrual cycles. In 1980, researchers discovered that the pheromones responsible for this menstrual synchrony are present in underarm perspiration.

Between 1975 and 1986, Dr. Winnifred Cutler and her colleagues at the University of Pennsylvania and later at Stanford University investigated multiple functions of pheromones in human sexual physiology and behavior. Dr. Cutler's group conducted seminal experiments demonstrating that human pheromones play a significant role in the relationship between women's reproductive cycles and their sexual behavior.

Most of us exposed to the general fund of scientific knowledge processed by the media have at least heard of pheromones—but we have had far less opportunity to learn about something known as the Major Histocompatability Complex, or MHC. A group of Swiss researchers in the department of immunology at the University of Bern describes the MHC as "an immunologically important group of genes that appear to be under natural as well as sexual selection."

What this boils down to is that each of us inherits genes that have at least two sets of powerful functions:

• **To influence body odors and body-odor preferences in humans, which is an inborn basis of
attraction between the sexes;**

and, at the same time,

• **To determine the inborn constitution and
thresholds of our immune system.**

Clinical research shows that the MHC is nature's elegant
and ingenious way of influencing a woman to be attracted to
a man who has a package of immunity-determining genes that
will maximize the couple's likelihood of being fertile, of car-
rying pregnancy through to term, and of bearing healthy and
immunologically well-equipped children. The functions of the
MHC genes, when free to operate as designed by nature, have
implications for our species' capacity to adapt to evolving challenges to our immune systems.

Of key importance to our understanding of the risks of
menstrual suppression is a finding, by the Swiss researchers, that
a woman's preference for a male with a particular MHC
depends on her hormonal status. For this study, researchers cat-
egorized male and female students into three distinguishable
MHC "types." Each male student wore a T-shirt for two con-
secutive nights. The next day, each female student was asked to
rate the odors of six T-shirts. The women scored the male
body odors as more pleasant when they differed from the men
in their own MHC than when they were more similar.
However, *the difference in odor assessment and preference was
radically altered when the women rating the odors were taking
oral contraceptives.*

A hot-off-the-press publication in the journal *Nature Genetics* reports that women are most enduringly attracted to men whose MHC-determined odors are neither identical to their own nor completely unfamiliar. Since the MHC genes are responsible BOTH for determining the thresholds and varieties of immune mechanisms of an individual AND for establishing pheromonal "types" that affect partner choice, nature has provided that a woman is normally attracted to a man with an *optimally different* package of immune equipment from her own. The disruption of women's natural hormonal cycle through the use of oral contraceptives has consequences to their personal lives and potential implications for the future well-being of the human species.

An article in *New Science* magazine, "Scent of a Man," by Alison Motluk, draws attention to the subject of pheromones as the basis of attraction. She refers to a poll taken by Rachel Herz from Brown University in Providence, Rhode Island, who asked 166 women "about what makes a man attractive—specifically, attractive enough to go to bed with." Ms. Herz found that "out of a variety of factors, including appearance, the sound of his voice and how his skin feels, women respondents said that a man's scent was **paramount.**"

Given the fact that a woman's use of oral contraceptives changes her response to MHC-determined male scent, Ms. Herz suggests to women on the Pill who think they've met "Mr. Right" to change to another method of birth control for a while, to "see if you're still attracted." This sounds like engaging Ph.D. thesis material to me.

Attraction is not the only consequence of nature-designed MHC pairing. Optimal MHC compatibility dramatically improves the likelihood of a couple's fertility and the prospect of the woman's giving birth to healthy offspring. Dr. Carole

Ober and her group of geneticists and anthropologists at the University of Chicago have conducted a series of landmark studies demonstrating that couples whose MHC genes are "too similar" are at increased risk for problems with fertility, miscarriage, and babies born with physical impairments. Since it appears that women using oral contraceptives are most attracted to men whose MHC genes are similar to their own, these factors are worrisome.

In 1960, the year that the FDA approved the use of the Pill, its pheromonal, genetic, immunological, and reproductive implications were unknown. Scientific and medical research reveals, day by day, more of the astounding complexity of our human physiology. We know some of the dangers of menstrual suppression, but we cannot, today, imagine them all. Remember some of the headlines and comments in support of menstrual suppression?

I think we have to disabuse health professionals and women of the idea that monthly menstruation is natural, normal and healthy.

We're into the era of medicine making life more convenient.

Nuisance or natural and healthy: Should monthly menstruation be optional for women?

Continuous use of ordinary oral contraceptives safely lets women control . . . whether and when they choose to bleed. When such a safe, simple, and inexpensive treatment is already so widely available, women should not have to be driven loony by their lunar cycles if they prefer not to bleed each month.

No More Period. Period.

Unless you're trying to get pregnant, there's no physiological reason to have a monthly period.

There's really no good medical reason for menstruation.

"Nuisance?" "Convenience?" "Expense?"

What we don't know CAN hurt us, in ways and to extents that we cannot even imagine. The potential cost of manipulating women's hormonal chemistry for the sake of convenience brings to mind my favorite bumper sticker:

So you think education is expensive?
Try IGNORANCE.

Chapter 3

The Iron
Hypothesis

A remarkable and, until now, largely unrecognized physiological *benefit* comes to us, women, *because* we bleed every month.

Research is showing that menstruation prevents some degree of arteriosclerotic changes in the walls of blood vessels, protecting us from increased risks of heart attacks and strokes.

More than twenty years ago, in the *Lancet* of June 13, 1981, Dr. Jerome L. Sullivan, of the University of Florida College of Medicine, went on record with the following innovative statement:

> *I propose the hypothesis that the greater incidence of heart disease in men and postmenopausal women compared with the incidence*

in premenopausal women results from **higher levels of stored iron** *in the two groups.*

Sullivan suggested, in other words, that monthly blood loss protects menstruating women against heart disease. Imagine this poster material for blood donation drives:

DONATING BLOOD, REGULARLY, CAN PROTECT YOUR HEART

Nature has provided women, during our reproductive years, with a natural protective mechanism about which few of us know. While we've heard a lot about "iron-deficiency anemia," and we know that we need enough iron in our diets to keep ourselves healthy, we know considerably less about the risks of excessive amounts of stored iron. Few of us have any idea how iron-rich our diets may be.

Do you know, for example, that three-quarters of one cup of "enriched" breakfast cereal supplies a full day's recommended daily allowance (RDA) of iron (18 milligrams) for women of menstrual age, and is an amount that *exceeds* the RDA for males of any age and for females of other ages— amounts that range from 7 mg per day to 11 mg per day? Recommended dietary iron for men and women age fifty-one and older is about 8 to 10 mg per day. Only pregnant women are advised to take in more iron—27 mg per day. Even nursing mothers' iron needs are met by a diet that provides 9 to 10 mg of iron per day.

Fundamental to understanding Dr. Sullivan's "iron hypothesis" is the following fact:

Iron is an essential nutrient **for which there is no nat-**

ural mechanism other than menstruation though which our body can excrete excess accumulation.

Dr. Sullivan pointed out that:

- Patients with diseases in which their bodies accumulate iron are known to develop heart failure.
- Men accumulate stored iron in the years following their adolescence.
- Menopausal women who do not use hormonal therapy to bleed cyclically accumulate stored iron to levels found in men, and *in rough proportion to their added risk of developing heart disease.*
- High-fiber diets retard iron absorption (one way in which fiber may help protect against cardiovascular disease).

Dr. Sullivan emphasized that, in parts of the world where the population suffers from iron deficiency on the basis of inadequate diet or parasitic disease, the types of heart disease that kill large numbers of American men are rare. In fact, among undernourished and iron-deficient men, it is not uncommon to find rates of heart disease that are lower than those of young American women.

In 1989, the *American Heart Journal* published Dr. Sullivan's substantial paper, with a description of some of the complex mechanisms (involving antioxidants and iron-dependent enzymes) through which stored iron might damage the cardio-vascular system, and where he further observes the following:

- Aspirin may help in preventing heart attacks, in part, by reducing stored iron as a result of mild gastric irritation and microscopic blood loss.

- Young women who regularly take oral contraceptives that reduce their monthly bleed may have levels of stored iron usually seen in older, perimenopausal women—*which contributes to their increased risk for cardiovascular disease.*
- Women who have had a hysterectomy (*including young women*) and postmenopausal women (neither of whom have monthly blood loss) have increased levels of stored iron—*which contributes to their increased risk for cardiovascular disease.*

In 1996, the *Journal of Clinical Epidemiology* published Dr. Sullivan's provocative paper "Iron Versus Cholesterol—Perspectives on the Iron and Heart Disease Debate"—in which he proposes that high serum cholesterol is a *weaker risk factor* for cardiovascular disease than is stored iron. While Sullivan **does** identify elevated serum cholesterol as a significant cardiovascular risk factor, he emphasizes that stored iron is a **greater risk factor.** He raises several very interesting points:

- Cholesterol as "the villain" for cardiovascular disease is rigidly overemphasized and is too limited a focus.
- Cholesterol-lowering drugs are definitely not without serious risks. More attention should be paid to boosting the body's antioxidant defenses, since *"the available evidence suggests that even a large increase in plasma cholesterol may do no harm **so long as the body's antioxidant defenses are sufficiently enhanced.**"*

Dr. Sullivan draws attention to a genetically inherited metabolic disorder of cholesterol metabolism that has a mouthful of a name: familial hypercholesterolemia. Women who inherit this condition, even when they are quite young, have cholesterol levels of 600 milligrams per deciliter! This is more than three times what is considered to be the upper limit of "acceptable" to the cholesterol-watchers and our doctors. Sullivan points out that there is a "remarkably low incidence of clinically apparent heart disease in young women *as long as they are menstruating.*" Young men who suffer from this genetic disorder, and whose cholesterol levels may actually be somewhat lower than the women's, ARE found to be at increased risk for heart attacks and strokes.

After women with these astronomically high levels of cholesterol go through menopause, their risk of cardiovascular disease increases dramatically. Dr. Sullivan explains that *the young women (with extraordinarily high cholesterol levels) are protected from the development of heart disease as long as they continue to lose excess iron through regular menstrual bleeding.*

By 1998, Dr. Sullivan was not a lone voice on the subject of stored iron as a cardiovascular risk factor. Several papers, including important studies by two sets of researchers in Finland and in Austria, had demonstrated that increased levels of stored iron are linked to the early development of atherosclerosis in men. In 1999, an impressive review of the research *pro-* and *con-* the iron hypothesis was published in the *Archives of Internal Medicine,* affirming that "strong epidemiological evidence is available that iron is an important factor in the process of atherosclerosis." Concerns about men's cardiovascular risk have, in recent decades, received impressive research and clinical attention, with impressively beneficial results.

Both gender-limited research and clinical neglect have been contributing to the fact that women's cardiovascular health is becoming an increasingly serious problem. Studies have been done *measuring* stored iron in menopausal women, all noting in their descriptive sections that increased iron stores have been shown to increase cardiovascular risk. However, I was unable to find a single study designed to evaluate the specific risk to *women's* cardiovascular health of increased iron stores—not one study that parallels the Finnish and the Austrian studies of the risk to men.

In 2000, authors of an article published in *The Journal of Women's Health and Gender-Based Medicine* entitled "Improved Iron Status Parameters May Be a Benefit of Hormone Replacement Therapy" did not evaluate the women's iron parameters in relation to cardiovascular risk, but did nicely sum up a description of the complex mechanisms believed to underlie the relationship of stored iron to cardiovascular disease:

- Serum ferritin (the protein that carries iron) is a measure of total body iron stores.
- When storage is overloaded, iron binding becomes saturated, leaving free (unbound) iron.
- Free iron has the potential to increase free radical production and trigger the oxidation of low-density-lipoprotein (LDL) cholesterol, (which) leads to foam cell generation, atherosclerosis, and coronary heart disease.

"Foam cell generation," "atherosclerosis," "coronary heart disease" . . . sounds bad. These are the consequences of the buildup of excess stored iron, iron that women's bodies are designed naturally to regulate through normal menstruation.

Encouraging young women to stop menstruating without monitoring and regulating the increased levels of

stored iron portends to have serious consequences in terms of women's early development of cardiovascular disease, heart attacks, and strokes.

The information on prevention of these diseases with which we are most familiar refers to antioxidants—foods and vitamins that are good for our hearts by reducing "free radical" production. (I can't help associating "free radicals" with out-of-control wildfolk of the 1960s.) In researching the role of stored iron in the development of atherosclerosis (the buildup of fatty and calcium-hardened material in the linings of arteries), what I've learned about antioxidants and free radicals has increased my appreciation for the potential benefits of eating foods rich in antioxidants. As we approach and pass menopause, we can fight these "free radicals" by using antioxidant vitamin supplements in recommended safe dosage.

Among the fruits of my exploration into foods high in antioxidant capacity (measured in "oxygen radical absorbance capacity," or ORAC units) was learning that, of all foods, *prunes* rank highest—providing 5,770 ORAC units per 100 grams (about seven prunes) as compared with broccoli, which has a relatively meager 890 ORAC units per 100 grams (one cup). Since prunes are also high in fiber, and so decrease iron absorption from the diet, it appears that my Auntie Rosie was on to something even better than she knew with those prunes!

Here, where we concern ourselves with the potential risks of tampering with the natural order, is a fitting place for another particular discovery I made in the course of my research: The consequences of manipulating our natural body chemistry, even in the form of what we may have been advised is "moderate" vitamin supplementation, can do significant harm.

I was surprised and disturbed to learn that supplementation

with retinol, the common form of Vitamin A found in animal foods (such as fish oils and liver) accelerates the process of bone loss, osteoporosis, and hip fractures. In this regard, cod liver oil is NOT a good idea. Beta-carotene, the form of Vitamin A found in vegetables and fruits, is clearly a safer supplement.

What's more, it doesn't take a megadosage of Vitamin A from fish oil to do harm. An article in the January 2, 2002, issue of the *Journal of the American Medical Association* reports that women who consumed 3,000 micrograms of Vitamin A in retinol form (equivalent to about 10,000 IU of Vitamin A) "had a significantly increased risk of hip fracture."

Looking at the label of my own bottle of Vitamin A supplement, I am alarmed to see that it has 25,000 IU of Vitamin A, derived from "fish liver oil." I had thought that 25,000 IU of this antioxidant was a good thing, but now I'm relieved that I haven't been taking it all regularly. Since many of our foods are "fortified" by the addition of vitamins, commonly including Vitamin A in the form of retinol, we may be ingesting significantly more retinol than we realize.

Nutritionists are advising that it is safest to obtain the antioxidant benefits of Vitamin A through moderate consumption of carrots, sweet potato, and dried apricots—excellent sources of the beta-carotene form. As a natural consequence of eating a moderate and balanced diet, using safe vitamin supplements, and allowing the regular depletion of stored iron through normal, regular menstruation, the cells of a woman's body are given their best protection from those free radicals.

Consistent with the bias in his book promoting menstrual suppression, Dr. Elsimar Coutinho is dismissive of the growing body of information we have implicating stored iron as a cardiovascular risk factor. Instead, he emphasizes the benefits of menstrual suppression to women in Third World countries who suffer from iron deficiency anemia!

Can we take seriously Dr. Coutinho's suggestion that an acceptable approach to iron deficiency caused by inadequate diet and intestinal parasites is to dose undernourished women with pharmaceutical drugs in order to prevent further iron loss through menstruation? Women in miserable circumstances deserve attention both to wholesome diet and to decent health care and safe birth control.

So long as the information is available, those of us who are fortunate to have abundant options can make informed choices. Now we can add to what we know about vitamin supplementation, exercise, and diet the growing body of information pointing to the probability that the monthly bleed is a blessing to the balance of iron in our bodies and makes an important contribution to our health and longevity.

Chapter 4

The Blind Men and the Elephant

Since the publication of *The Hormone of Desire,* which focuses on the role of testosterone in female physiology, women quite regularly contact me for consultation to learn and evaluate the options for help with their hormonal problems. A few months ago, I received the following letter from a very unhappy young woman. With her permission, given in the hope that it might help other women, I reprint it here:

Subj: PLEASE HELP!
Date: 9/24/01 10:13:44 P.M. Eastern Daylight Time
Hello:
 My name is _____ and I am 24 years old. I am cur-rently on Depo-Provera and am very unhappy with what it has done to me. I am in _____, California, and have an excellent physician, only she is very hard to get an appointment with,

sometimes it takes months, and I only get to see a physician's assistant. I don't necessarily feel comfortable with that. My OB didn't offer me any knowledge on what this drug may do to my desire for sex. I am sorry to bother you on the Internet so randomly like this, but I am at the bottom of the barrel [sic] and it just so happened that Depo-Provera and its effects came to be in my textbook, "Our Sexuality," where your book is referenced a lot. I just need a guiding hand.

After having my baby two years ago, we decided that I would finish college and we would save before we had another baby. I read about many different kinds of birth control, and then a friend told me about the Depo-Provera shot. Every 3 months sounded great to me. I have since received 2 shots and my 3rd is scheduled for October but I am DEFINITELY not going to get it again. I know that I am too young for menopause, but I am suffering from certain things and wonder if hormone replacement therapy could help me right now. I am experiencing 4 of the symptoms described in my text that you wrote in your book: "Decrease in one's customary level of sexual desire; Reduced sensitivity of the genitals and the nipples to sexual stimulation; Overall reduction in general levels of sexual arousability, possibly accompanied by decreased orgasmic capacity and/or less intense orgasms." And I also experience the last symptom: "Diminished energy levels."

In my class textbook it mentions that because I am taking Depo-Provera, my testosterone levels are at almost nothing. It also states that, like in men, women also need testosterone for sexual desire.

I am in need of any kind of help you can give me. I have spoken to my OB/GYN, whose only advice to me was to plan a date or dinner with my husband and try to make it romantic.

My problem is not whether I can make a romantic moment happen; it's whether I am going to feel like being romantic at all. My husband is growing frustrated with me and it is hindering our relationship with each passing day.

I feel betrayed that none of the physicians or assistants I have talked to ever mentioned what Depo-Provera actually was—that it is sometimes administered to sex offenders and that it can make you have no desire for sex at all. I also wasn't told that it was used for prostate cancer and other diseases. I feel as if I wasn't given enough information to go on, and I hope that other women are not going through what I am, because it isn't fair. I am just trying to go back to normal and have the relationship with my husband go back to the loving way that it was. I miss my sexuality.

Not only did I go from 100% desire to 0%, but I also am much more tired then [sic] I used to be. I do exercise at least 5 times a week, and I am trying my best to be knowledgeable about my body and my needs. I just want someone to tell me there is something that I can do to help get my desire back. I don't even like to be touched anymore. I find that hard to deal with, and it is bothering me emotionally.

If you can refer me to a California physician or someone I can just talk to who can tell me something I can do, that would be amazing. I am so desperate.

(signed _____)

I recognized from her letter that this young woman was experiencing the disturbing consequences to her hormonal balance resulting from the use of Depo-Provera, a synthetic progestin injected about once every three months for the purpose of birth control, and presented as having the added "benefit" of "no periods." It is the drug promoted by Dr. Elsimar Coutinho (author of *Is Menstruation Obsolete?*) as beneficial and largely innocuous.

All too frequently, women are injected with Depo-Provera without forewarning about its potential side effects and disturbing risks, which include initial bleeding and spotting, headaches, abdominal bloating, nausea, constipation, depression, irritability, fatigue, mood changes, breast pain and engorgement, varicose veins, loss of sex drive, painful intercourse, hot flashes, dry vagina, extended infertility, detrimental alterations in blood cholesterol, and bone loss leading to the early development of osteoporosis. Once a woman has been injected with this drug, no matter how miserable she may be and no matter how severe her symptoms, she has to live with the effects for three months, until it has been "used up."

The woman whose letter we read suffered most bitterly from the impact of the drug on her body's available testosterone. Another method of menstrual suppression—which amounts to more or less nonstop use of oral contraceptives— also depresses testosterone levels. In order to understand this particular risk of menstrual suppression, we have to understand how testosterone works.

As I describe in *The Hormone of Desire:*

"What does testosterone do in a woman's body?"

Do you remember what it was like to begin to mature? It was testosterone that stimulated the growth of your pubic hair and underarm hair (there are testosterone receptors in the skin of the pubic area and in the skin of the underarm that are genetically programmed to react to testosterone by producing hair). And testosterone stimulated your skin to produce more oil, contributing to the acne of your early teenage years, but also the healthy glow of your skin and the shine of your hair.

In addition, there are testosterone receptors in the nipples of the developing breasts, as well as in the clitoris and in the vagina, which make them sensitive to sexual stimulation.

There are receptors *in the brain* that respond to testosterone by establishing the neurochemical basis for falling in love. . . . Without testosterone, we would have no pubic hair, decreased sensitivity to sexual pleasure in the nipples and genitals, and clearly decreased capacity to "turn on."

An endocrinologist's bible, the medical textbook *Reproductive Endocrinology,* edited by Drs. Samuel Yen and Robert Jaffe, states: "Testosterone and other androgens have some biological activity on virtually every tissue in the body." Testosterone works to keep the body functioning efficiently, making the best use of nourishment for growth and maintenance, and particularly contributing to the health of bones and muscles.

From the "kickoff" of testosterone production at puberty and as long as women have fully functioning ovaries, their bodies produce, on the average, three-tenths of one milligram of testosterone a day. Men's bodies produce more than twenty times as much, or an average of seven milligrams of testosterone per day.

A critical factor in understanding how menstrual suppression affects testosterone physiology for women requires knowing that testosterone is carried in the blood, most of it attached to a protein known as sex hormone binding globulin, or "SHBG." (My friend Jeanne's mnemonic for SHBG is "she big"—and "she big" is, certainly, a big problem.) Only a tiny amount of testosterone can remain unbound to this protein and "free" in the plasma—free to produce its effects on tissues.

Ninety-seven to ninety-nine percent of a woman's testosterone is attached to the immobilizing protein at any given time.

Only 1 percent to 3 percent of a woman's total testosterone is ever available to have its effect on tissues. Small changes in the production of SHBG can make a BIG difference in terms of libido, sexual sensitivity, and sexual pleasure.

Both estrogen and testosterone are carried on the same binding protein. Estrogen actually stimulates the production of *more* "she big," which then binds up still *more* of the testosterone, leaving less testosterone to be free to work on cells.

One point worth emphasizing is the fact that **the estrogen content even of "low dose" oral contraceptives is sufficient to stimulate the production of SHBG and to reduce the amount of available testosterone in a woman's body,** leading to troubling sexual side effects, reduced energy, and a diminished sense of well-being.

The use of Depo-Provera for birth control and menstrual suppression reduces available testosterone via a second mechanism: It reduces the production of testosterone by our ovaries. Ovarian tissue, which produces about half the body's testosterone, responds to stimulation by a pituitary hormone known as luteinizing hormone (LH). Depo-Provera effectively shuts down the pituitary's production of LH. That's a sure way to bottom out a woman's testosterone.

My earliest contact with the way hormones work happened in 1953, when I was fourteen and in ninth grade, and was allowed to drop Latin (oh happy day) in favor of Physiology and Health. Thrilled not to be translating *Caesar's Gallic Wars,* I learned with some pleasure a simplified scheme that explained the way that the pituitary gland (a gland that is part of the base of the brain) and the ovaries interact in women's reproductive physiology. That primitive explanation is now known to be incomplete at best and wrong at worst. But it is worth reviewing as a basis for appreciating the elegant refinements and the fact of their complexity that underlies the risks of disrupting the hormonal tapestry of the menstrual cycle.

Without an appreciation of the complexity of hormones' effects upon one another and of their far-reaching effects on every organ system in the body, we are not equipped to understand the risks of hormonal manipulation and disruption of the normal menstrual cycle.

With an appreciation of this complexity, we cannot be convinced that menstrual suppression is without detrimental effects and future risk.

What I was taught went something like this:

- We can consider a menstrual cycle to begin when our pituitary gland produces follicle-stimulating hormone (FSH), which signals the cells in the ovaries to grow, creating a sort of nest around a maturing egg. Many follicles with maturing eggs are stimulated to begin to grow each month, although only one egg may actually make it all the way to ovulation.
- The follicle cells produce estrogen, which, in turn, signals the cells lining the uterus to develop a bed of tissue rich in blood vessels (the endometrium), for potential planting of a fertilized egg.
- At about midway through the month of a "normal" menstrual cycle, estrogen levels are at their peak, and the mature egg pops out of the follicle and into the

oviduct, on its way into the uterus. In the intricate interplay of hormones, when the level of estrogen reaches a critical point, the pituitary stops producing FSH. Via a "feedback loop," the pituitary "reads" the level of estrogen and says, "We've got enough estrogen. We don't need any more. Cut off the FSH. Bring on the luteinizing hormone (LH)."

• The function of the LH produced by the pituitary is to stimulate the cells of the follicle that have been left behind to produce progesterone, whose important function in the menstrual cycle is to prepare and maintain the lining of the uterus (the endometrium) for implantation by a fertilized egg. After about two weeks, when the level of progesterone reaches a critical point, another feedback loop is activated, when the pituitary "reads" the level of progesterone and says, "We've got enough progesterone. We don't need any more. Cut off the LH."

When I was fourteen, the role of LH in stimulating testosterone production was never mentioned. In 1953, that was fully understandable. However, even in 2003, most physicians do not understand the critical function of LH and its implications. The consequence to women with normal ovaries whose production of LH is diminished for any reason—including the use of some birth control pills, Depo-Provera, or other similar hormone-manipulating pharmaceuticals, is potentially to suffer a compromised quality of life as a result of untreated testosterone deficiency.

• When an egg is fertilized and plants itself in the prepared lining of the womb, the cells of the growing placenta take over the job of producing the hormones that maintain the endometrial lining. If no fertilization and implantation have taken place, when the levels of progesterone produced by the ovary drop down, the lining of the uterus begins to shed. About four weeks from start of the FSH to finish of the LH and, voila!— a menstrual period.

When I learned this sequence, back in the '50s, I thought that it was a little complicated but pretty neat.

In 1962, when I was in medical school, I learned about another layer to the hormonal underpinnings of the menstrual cycle. Drs. Ernst and Berta Scharrer taught our courses in neuroanatomy and neurophysiology. The Scharrers were husband and wife pioneering researchers who, though not Jewish, left Germany in 1937 for the United States because of the Nazi policies against their Jewish colleagues. (An anecdote about their life in wartime Germany, told at the time of Berta's death, in 1995: "Berta described that they often came to work with briefcases in both hands so they wouldn't have to give the 'heil Hitler' business.")

Well—the Scharrers had made groundbreaking discoveries showing that the pituitary's production of FSH and LH was regulated by "releasing factors" produced by the hypothalamus of the brain, factors that are, themselves, regulated by levels of estrogen and progesterone produced in the ovaries. This complex of hormonal interactions was known as "the hypophyseal portal system."

I remember the drama of Dr. Ernst Scharrer's beginning one neuroanatomy lecture by cradling in his surgical-gloved hands a specimen of a preserved human brain, ascending the stairway of the amphitheater where we sat for our lectures, and saying, with evident respect, "Here is an example of matter contemplating itself."

Advances in knowledge of neuroendocrinology are such that today, sixty years since the Scharrers' early work, a full description of the hormonal regulation of the menstrual cycle is mind-boggling. Let me quote a section from one of the more lucid texts that explains something now known as the "two-cell system"—describing how two kinds of cells in the egg follicles of the ovaries, "theca cells" and "granulosa cells," are involved in the sequence of hormonal events of the menstrual cycle.

I include this section **not** with the aim of shedding light on the **substance** of what is now known about the hormonal regulation of the menstrual cycle, but with the aim of demonstrating the complexity of the factors involved. Hold on to your seat and read fast. There will be no quiz at the end of the section.

- FSH receptors are present on the granulosa cells.
- FSH receptors are induced by FSH itself.
- LH receptors are present on the theca cells and initially absent on the granulosa cells, but, as the follicle grows, FSH induces the appearance of LH receptors on the granulosa cells.
- FSH induces aromatase enzyme activity in granulosa cells.
- The above actions are modulated by autocrine and paracrine factors secreted by the theca and granulosa cells.

The textbook goes on to explain:

The regulation of FSH receptors on granulosa cells is relatively complex. (**You can say THAT again!**) *Although FSH increases the activity of its own receptor gene in a cyclic AMP-mediated mechanism, this action is influenced by inhibitory agents, such as epidermal growth factor, fibroblast growth factor, and even a gonadotropin-releasing hormone (GnRH)-like protein. Inhibin and activin are produced in the granulosa in response to FSH, and activin has the important autocrine role of enhancing FSH actions, especially the production of FSH receptors. . . .*

EGAD.

There is *one* statement that follows this section of the text that is pretty straightforward, and clearly complicates what I was taught in ninth grade:

> *. . . estrogen secretion by the follicle prior to ovulation is the result of combined LH and FSH stimulation. . . .*

Evidently FSH and LH aren't turned "on" and "off" nicely in sequence. So much for that neat "feedback loop" theory.

The increasingly complex and growing body of knowledge on the subject of hormonal function demonstrates that estrogen, progesterone, and testosterone have effects not only on the tissues and organs concerned with reproduction, but also on virtually every organ system in the body. Some of these effects, such as estrogen's effect to preserve bone density, and testosterone's effect—via a different mechanism—to build new bone, are clearly recognized at this time. We know enough now to know that manipulation of the hormonal milieu affects not only the levels of the hormone(s) supplied, but also the levels and tissue effects of other hormones and regulators, with far-reaching, potentially undesirable (even unpredictable) consequences.

Without an appreciation of the complexity of hormones' effects upon one another and of their far-reaching effects on every organ system in the body, we are not equipped to understand the risks of hormonal manipulation and disruption of the normal menstrual cycle.

With an appreciation of this complexity, we cannot be convinced that menstrual suppression is without detrimental effects and future risk.

In the case of the woman who wrote to me about her messed-up sex life following Depo-Provera injections for birth control and menstrual suppression, her consequences were, with our present state of knowledge, predictable. Here's the scoop.

The "depo" of Depo-Provera means that the synthetic progestin was mixed with an oil that, when injected into her muscle, created a kind of reservoir of the hormone designed to diffuse into her bloodstream over the next three months. The level of progestin in her blood circulation came NOT from her ovaries but from the injected drug and was "read" by all the neuroendocrine elements in the cells of her brain and ovaries as though it had been produced by her own ovaries.

Through complex feedback mechanisms, the levels of progestin supplied by the injection cut back her body's production BOTH of FSH and of LH—which stopped eggs from maturing in her ovaries, clearly preventing the possibility of pregnancy. Depo-Provera is definitely an effective contraceptive.

However, reducing both FSH and LH had other, less desirable consequences in her body. Since her ovaries needed LH to stimulate their production of testosterone, this unfortunate woman wound up with testosterone deficiency—which generated the sexual problems that troubled her. The combination of FSH and LH suppression by Depo-Provera also cut back her ovaries' production of estrogen, which gave this young woman menopausal symptoms of hot flashes and dry vagina. Moreover, she had not been told that, if she continued to use Depo-Provera, the lowered estrogen levels would eventually lead to bone loss and put her at risk for early osteoporosis.

Both estrogen and testosterone have effects essential to women's health, including the maintenance of the strength of bones, the lubrication of the tissues of the vagina, and the balance of brain chemistry that affects mood and prevents depression. In fact, estrogen can legitimately be considered a "natural antidepressant." It regulates neurotransmitters in the brain and keeps the level of one particularly important enzyme, monoamine oxidase (MAO), in check. MAO is the enzyme that metabolizes serotonin, a neurochemical with powerful effects on mood.

Let's look at this other example of a cascade of effects that reproductive hormones can generate. Stick with it. While the explanation has some complexity, I believe that you can get your mind around this one without a full case of "the boggles."

- The lower the level of estrogen we have, the higher the level of MAO.
- The higher the level of MAO, the lower the level of serotonin.
- The lower the level of serotonin, the more depressed a woman will be.

Prozac, Zoloft, Paxil, Celexa, and the other "SSRI's"—
"**S**elective **S**erotonin **R**e-uptake **I**nhibitors"—lighten depression by maintaining higher levels of serotonin in the brain via a mechanism that slows its "reuptake" by receptors. While often effective in treating depression, these drugs have unfortunate side effects that interfere with sexual libido and response. Equally unfortunate is the ignorance of many health-care providers about the "natural antidepressant" effects of estrogen and testosterone. Too often, depressed postmenopausal women and women who have had a hysterectomy and would benefit from responsible, low-dose hormone supplementation are instead prescribed an SSRI, which compounds their sexual difficulties and may not even help their depression.

As true for me today as it was when I wrote this final paragraph of *The Hormone of Desire* seven years ago:

> *I will affirm what has always been and still remains my personal practice where tampering with the natural order is concerned: Do as little as you can and as much as you need, and no one knows better than you.*

No one knows better than you, that is, provided that you

- Believe what your body tells you;

and

- Learn what you can from reliable sources about available options for "tampering with the natural order" and of the potential benefits *and risks* of using them.

The risk of holding to one theory and approach to hormone supplementation or to the safety of menstrual suppression as "THE" way to go, is the possibility of operating rather like the blind men and the elephant. Based on a Chinese parable that originated during the Han dynasty (202 B.C.–A.D. 220) and was later expanded in India, this poem by American poet and Vermont lawyer John Godfrey Saxe (1816–1887) demonstrates, with wit and charm, his attraction to the value of a full and balanced perspective—a characteristic that was no doubt useful in his work as attorney, editor, and politician.

The Blind Men and the Elephant

It was six men of Indostan
To learning much inclined
Who went to see the Elephant
(Though all of them were blind),
That each by observation
Might satisfy his mind.

The First approached the Elephant,
And happening to fall
Against his broad and sturdy side,
At once began to bawl:
"God bless me! but the Elephant
Is very like a wall!"

The Second, feeling of the tusk
Cried, "Ho! what have we here,
So very round and smooth and sharp?
To me 'tis mighty clear
This wonder of an Elephant
Is very like a spear!"

The Third approached the animal,
And happening to take
The squirming trunk within his hands,
Thus boldly up he spake:
"I see," quoth he, "the Elephant
Is very like a snake!"

The Fourth reached out an eager hand,
And felt about the knee:
"What most this wondrous beast is like
Is mighty plain," quoth he;
"'Tis clear enough the Elephant
Is very like a tree!"

The Fifth, who chanced to touch the ear,
Said: "E'en the blindest man
Can tell what this resembles most;
Deny the fact who can,
This marvel of an Elephant
Is very like a fan!"

The Sixth no sooner had begun
About the beast to grope,
Than, seizing on the swinging tail
That fell within his scope,
"I see," quoth he, "the Elephant
Is very like a rope!"

And so these men of Indostan
Disputed loud and long,
Each in his own opinion
Exceeding stiff and strong,

Though each was partly in the right,
And all were in the wrong!

Moral:

So oft in theologic wars,
The disputants, I ween,
Rail on in utter ignorance
Of what each other mean,
And prate about an Elephant
Not one of them has seen!

The women who contact me about their hormonal problems have reinforced my sense that women are as similar to and as different from one another as snowflakes—having a common fundamental identity and no two the same. Some (estimated at 15 to 20 percent—not nearly as many as wish) women "breeze through" menopause without even thinking of needing hormonal supplements. About 15 to 20 percent have a really tough time with the menopausal transition, which can smooth out several years after the last menstrual period—often with the help of careful hormone supplementation. The remaining 60 to 70 percent fall somewhere between these two extremes.

About 50 percent of menopausal women (and some percentage of women in the years leading up to menopause) experience a significant loss of available testosterone, with detrimental effects to sexual libido, sensitivity, and response. Not all women are troubled by it.

Following her menopause, Gloria Steinem, in an interview published in June 1999, described herself as being quite at peace with her loss of sexual libido and with having become celibate:

With myself, since menopause, that part of my brain that had always been a reliable home for sex is gone. It's gone! If I had heard myself say this 20 years ago, I would have heard it as a loss. But it isn't. It's fine. . . . Not better or worse, just different.

Interviewed by Barbara Walters on *20/20* less than two years later—after, at age sixty-six, she had met and partnered in marriage (for the first time) with a man she loves—Ms. Steinem acknowledged that her sexual interest had sparked up again. The revitalization certainly did appear to be quite delightful to her. Asked for her comment on this development, Ms. Steinem ventured: "Well—well, I think—I think that perhaps the truth is that behavior creates hormones, just as hormones create behavior."

While not a universal truth, there is something to her idea. We know that sexual activity has a small stimulating effect on testosterone production, more for women(!) than for men. Some women do find, to their distinct pleasure, that a new relationship "primes the pump" well enough. Others, though, find that sexual libido lost as a function of aging persists as a problem in spite of having a new (or old) attractive and loving partner. Many women who contact me for help have younger male partners and are concerned about their own lack of sexual interest and response. The complexity of internal and external chemistry cannot be denied.

Today's crop of books on menopause includes those advocating one or another particular approach to the constellation of symptoms that challenge, to a greater or lesser degree, most perimenopausal and postmenopausal women. As much as we might like to believe it could be so, the idea that one hormonal approach "fits all" or even MOST women is simply not true.

From my appreciation of the interplay of hormones and the complexity of hormonal effects throughout the body, I am uneasy about any approach to hormone supplementation that departs radically from the balances of hormones that occur naturally in our fertile years.

Advocates of the use of natural progesterone cream as the sole supplement wherever possible for women from age thirty to ninety who have problems referable to "hormone imbalance" are advising such a departure. The most potentially worrisome aspect of steady progesterone supplementation is the possibility that it might increase the risk of breast cancer. A Swedish study published in 1989 observes that the greatest proliferation of breast tissue cells during a normal menstrual cycle coincides with the time of maximum progesterone production. Their study, along with publications by a group of researchers at the University of Southern California, Los Angeles, gives statistical support to the possibility that progesterone may be a risk factor for breast cancer.

The risk/benefit analysis of progesterone use is complex. Since estrogen supplemental therapy can stimulate the tissue lining the uterus, with the potential of increased risk of endometrial cancer, physicians who prescribe estrogen supplementation to menopausal women customarily prescribe some regimen of progestin to keep endometrial growth in check.

The group at USC emphasizes that breast cancer is more dangerous than is endometrial cancer. This same group also warns about estrogen's being a risk factor for breast cancer, and have published reports suggesting that women with a strong family history of breast cancer are at substantially greater risk if they use oral contraceptives. They are investigating ways to shut down the menstrual cycle completely at the level of the pituitary gland, to induce menopause in younger women, and to "add back" bits of hormones to combat symptoms of deficiency.

Such radical intervention might theoretically be a reasonable choice for women at extreme genetic risk for breast cancer or ovarian cancer, and for whom osteoporosis, cardiovascular risks, mood alterations, and the rest of the effects of hormone manipulation we have been considering take second place to a very high probability that they will, early in their lives, die from breast cancer or ovarian cancer. Each woman presents a unique constellation of risk factors, and a unique challenge for risk/benefit evaluation of hormonal supplementation or manipulation.

A constellation of factors, such as number and competence of hormone receptors, levels of binding proteins, enzyme levels, other health factors, medications, genetic predispositions, relationship issues, environmental factors, and life-stress levels all contribute to the complexity and variation of response to hormonal intervention from woman to woman. "The Whole Elephant" of hormonal chemistry has an incredibly large number of aspects.

Publications in the medical literature on the subject of progesterone cream range from reports of women "overdosing" with progesterone cream to studies showing that even two to four times the manufacturer's recommended amount of Pro-gest cream (one teaspoonful morning and night) does not provide levels of progesterone sufficient to protect the lining of the uterus from developing cancerous changes that can be caused by the use of supplementary estrogen.

On another topic of controversy: A recent study by researchers in the United Kingdom, published in the October 2001 *British Medical Journal,* showed that "progesterone is ineffective" in alleviating the symptoms of PMS. Theories about the cause of PMS range from "too much estrogen and not enough progesterone," to "too much progesterone and not enough estrogen," to something about "prostaglandins," and on and on. Researchers at the National Institutes for Health (NIH) have shown that women with premenstrual syndrome have "normal hormonal changes" during the menstrual cycle. They concluded that abnormal levels of cycling hormones do not cause PMS, which they consider to be "an abnormal response—deterioration in mood state—in susceptible women."

The blind men and the elephant, again. "Susceptible women?" The NIH study demonstrates the limits of what we know about the effects of the complex hormonal constitutions that vary from woman to woman. Of course no *one* approach to the symptoms of PMS works for all women who suffer them. A small dose of Zoloft (sertraline)—as little as 25 mg—taken for a few days ONLY can help some women's premenstrual moods and shifts without wreaking havoc on their sexual interests and responses. (I've also seen a few days' use of Zoloft to counterbalance the symptoms that for many menopausal women accompany the progestin part of their hormone supplementation.) Still, Zoloft doesn't help everybody. And it's no surprise to me that while some women report that natural progesterone cream helps their symptoms of PMS, others report otherwise.

The "natural progesterone advocates" emphasize the fact that *synthetic* progestins can cause an array of problematic symptoms. For the most part, they play down the difficulties that women can have with the use of natural progesterone. I have observed that, in the presence of normal range levels of estrogen, supplemental natural progesterone does cause fewer problems than do synthetic progestins—but only for some women.

I wish it weren't the case, but the truth is that natural progesterone is not without potential undesirable—and sometimes intolerable—side effects. After menopause, many women find the most disturbing effects of supplemental natural progesterone to be depression and fatigue. Postmenopausal women with an intact uterus who benefit from supplemental estrogen (and must use a progestin to avoid overstimulation of the uterine lining with subsequent increased risk of endometrial cancer) sometimes have a very tough time finding a tolerable progesterone regimen. Natural progesterone is no panacea.

Today, in evaluating consequences to women of hormone manipulation, with all that we know, we have yet to know the full scope and the long-term effects of reproductive hormones on other organ systems.

As this book goes to press, August 2002, media headlines have instigated chaos and confusion for menopausal women taking hormone supplemental therapy. In response to the front page *New York Times* story reporting, misinterpreting, and distorting the implications of the interruption of one "arm" of the Women's Health Initiative (a large, federally funded study of the long-term effects on menopausal women of combined estrogen/synthetic progesterone treatment), my letter was published on July 18, 2002:

> *To the Editor:*
> *What has been tested and found risky is one particular drug, Prempro, a pharmaceutical that combines conjugated estrogen with a synthetic progestin.*
> *Unfortunately, the study made no provision to follow*

the risks to women of supplemental estrogen in combination with natural progesterone on an intermittent cyclic basis, a regimen least likely to increase risks of breast cancer, heart attacks, and strokes.

Women should not be left thinking that all estrogen-progestin hormone replacement therapy is hazardous. What a pity that the study was poorly designed and that its conclusions lend themselves so well to misinterpretation.

Susan Rako, M.D.
Newtonville, Mass., July 9, 2002

Inflammatory headlines and feature stories appeared in newspapers, magazines, and on television news shows across the country (and, likely, abroad)—generalizing from the finding that *one particular hormone regimen had—ONCE AGAIN—been found to be potentially risky* to a warning that "(all) hormone therapy is dangerous." During the past decade, two acronymous studies, "PEPI" and "HERS," have provided some useful information, and, particularly with reference to the HERS study, have stirred substantial controversy. ("PEPI" stands for the Postmenopausal Estrogen/Progestin Interventions, and "HERS" for the Heart and Estrogen-progestin Replacement Study.) A recent editorial published in the journal *Circulation,* entitled "The Time Has Come to Stop Letting the HERS Tale Wag the Dogma," brilliantly addresses the misinterpretations and media hype that followed the publication of that study. The parallels between the response to the HERS study of 1998 and to the publication by the Women's Health Initiative in 2002 are unmistakable.

The complexity of issues that feed in to and confound

studies in women's reproductive health are painful to contemplate. Resistance and bias of every sort—psychological, political, economic, social—clutter the field and fight for dominance. I will leave the speculation to others, and do my best to lay out the recent history of research into the long-term effects—risks and benefits—of hormone supplemental therapy for menopausal women.

Significant welcome advance in knowledge about safe and effective hormone replacement therapy was achieved, in 1988, when the PEPI trial was designed to study the effects of estrogen/progestin regimens on heart disease risk factors and on the endometrium (the lining of the uterus). In particular, this study set out to compare the effects of estrogen alone and in combination with two different formulations of progestin. One of these formulations was "natural micronized progesterone" (MP) suspended in oil, which means natural progesterone that has been processed into very fine particles and mixed with oil for optimal absorption. MP was not yet available in the United States, but had been manufactured and prescribed for women in other parts of the world for some time. (MP has subsequently been approved by the FDA and, since 1999, has been available on prescription in the United States as Prometrium, manufactured by Solvay Pharmaceuticals.)

Based on "preliminary data" from other studies suggesting that, of all progestins, MP interferes *least* with estrogen's beneficial effects on cholesterol, the PEPI designers included a formulation of this natural progestin in their study. They decided, also, that women using both estrogen and progestin would follow a regimen of progestin dosage for only twelve days each month (cyclical use of progestin). The other progestin they studied, also on a cyclic basis, was Provera, the same synthetic progestin later chosen by the Women's Health Initiative for daily dosing. The decision by the designers of the PEPI trial to study the effects of cyclical natural micronized progesterone would prove to be very wise.

For use in the PEPI study, the pharmaceutical company Schering-Plough manufactured the micronized natural progesterone. Between December 1989 and February 1991, researchers recruited "875 healthy postmenopausal women aged 45 to 64 years" at seven clinical centers in the United States. Designed to run for three years, the study published its findings in 1995 and 1996—while the Women's Health Initiative trials were already well under way.

Between 1993 and 1998, the Women's Health Initiative (WHI) had enrolled 161,809 postmenopausal women in the age range of 50 to 79 years into a set of clinical trials at forty clinical centers in the United States. One of these trials studied the risks and benefits of a daily regimen of combined estrogen and synthetic progesterone. The study had been designed in 1991–1992, "using the accumulated evidence at the time." The WHI designers chose to study the effects of estrogen alone compared with only ONE formulation of progestin—the synthetic progestin, medroxyprogesterone acetate (Provera). They made the decision to test a combined formulation of conjugated equine estrogen (Premarin) together with Provera—a pharmaceutical known as Prempro. The decision of the designers of the WHI to study the effects only of the combined estrogen/synthetic progestin would ultimately result in the amputation of that "arm" of the study.

A serious problem presented itself earlier. The FIRST major disruption of the Women's Health Initiative occurred after the release of the PEPI trial results:

Women with an intact uterus and using estrogen without pro-gestin were at risk for developing cancer of the endometrium.

On the basis of this finding, in 1996, the section of the Women's Health Initiative of 331 women with an intact uterus who were being given estrogen without progestin was called to a halt. The prior year, in January 1995, the PEPI trial had already published its findings confirming that natural micronized pro-gesterone interfered *least* with the benefits to cholesterol provided by supplemental estrogen. It's a pity that the design-ers of the Women's Health Initiative could not, for whatever reasons, choose to test (and expand upon) the PEPI protocol by adding micronized natural progesterone to the estrogen, either daily or cyclically, for women in the WHI at risk in using estrogen alone. Instead, those women in the Women's Health Initiative were reassigned to the group of 7,771 women testing the effects of Prempro on a daily basis.

Two years later, in August 1998, the gong struck again. The results of the controversial HERS study were published. HERS was designed "to determine if estrogen plus progestin therapy alters the risk for coronary heart disease risks in post-menopausal women with established coronary disease." The effects of Prempro as compared with placebo were measured in a group totaling 2,763 women ranging in age from 55 to 79, and with an average age of 66.7. The study concluded not only that Prempro did NOT prevent heart attacks in these aging women who were already suffering from heart disease, but that, in the first year of the study, women using Prempro had an INCREASED incidence of blood clots, pulmonary embolism, and heart attacks.

The Women's Health Initiative took note of these findings, and, on the basis of "speculation that any early adverse effects of hormones on coronary heart disease (CHD) incidence was confined to women who have experienced prior CHD," elected to go on with their trial. In other words, the researchers at the Women's Health Initiative felt that it was safe to continue the study of Prempro on their population of menopausal and elderly women, who they believed NOT to be at undue risk because they were considered NOT to have preexisting heart disease.

Reviewing the report of the study by the Women's Health Initiative, I found that:

- Women in the study ranged in age from 50 to 79 years of age, with 66 percent of the women aged 60 to 79.
- Seventy-four percent of the women had NEVER used hormone supplements prior to enrolling in the study.

How wise was the decision to recruit a large majority of women who were ten to thirty years past menopause, sixty years of age or older at the start of the study, and about to take hormone supplements for the first time in their lives? Even "healthy" women aged 60 to 79 have aging arteries. In fact, more than one-third of the "healthy" women in the study had already been taking medication to control high blood pressure, 12 percent of the women had cholesterol levels requiring medication, 734 of the women were being treated for diabetes, 138 women had had a history of stroke, 472 women had a history of angina, and 296 women had had a prior heart attack. It appears that that's about what one can expect of a population of "healthy" aging women.

Looking further, I was not surprised to read that "drop-out rates [women who dropped out of the study] over time exceeded design projections, particularly early on [in the study]." The drug tested was Prempro, a pharmaceutical consisting of .625 mg of conjugated estrogen combined with 2.5 mg of Provera (an oral form of the same progestin used in Depo-Provera). While newly menopausal women, whose ovaries are still producing some estrogen, may tolerate synthetic progestin without too much difficulty, as women age and their estrogen levels drop off, more of them find that daily progestin makes them feel lousy. Even though, as the study reports, "some flexibility of the dosages of both estrogen and progestin was allowed to manage symptoms such as breast tenderness and vaginal bleeding," it is likely that some of the elderly women who had never before used estrogen supplementation found the conjugated estrogen not to be comfortable, either—causing symptoms of bloating, breast tenderness, nausea, and headaches. No wonder the "drop-out rate" was high early in the study!

More serious than discomfort, and the reason that this section of the WHI was stopped, was that more women using Prempro had heart attacks, strokes, and dangerous clots during the first few years of the study than did women using placebo. The authors of the HERS study reviewed in some details the various complex mechanisms by which progestin detrimentally affects the cardiovascular system, including its tendency to stimulate clot formation, to cause inflammatory reactions in the linings of blood vessels, and to interfere with the beneficial effects of estrogen on blood cholesterol.

Another group of women in the Women's Health Initiative, women who have had a hysterectomy and so do not need a progestin, has been testing the risks/benefits of estrogen alone. Since the number of dangerous events in that group has not exceeded the preset limits, that portion of the study continues.

What the Women's Health Initiative HAS shown is that Prempro—estrogen combined with synthetic progestin—not only will not prevent heart disease, but that its use itself may be a cardiovascular risk.

The event that precipitated the end of the Prempro trial in the Women's Health Initiative was the finding that, during the fifth and sixth years of the study, more women using Prempro developed invasive breast cancer than did women using placebo. The small increased risk of breast cancer in association with hormone supplementation is not a new observation. While estrogen has not been shown to *cause* breast cancer, estrogen can stimulate the growth of existing "estrogen sensitive" breast cancer. As we have discussed on page 73, some researchers implicate progesterone as a stimulant for breast cancer growth, noting that progesterone stimulates cell division in the breast. In addition, studies have shown that progesterone slows the clearance of estrogen, resulting in higher blood levels of estrogen for women using progesterone.

Since hormone levels and functions are complex and vary from woman to woman, hormone supplementation really must be individualized. Particularly with the limits of our knowledge of long-term effects, keeping blood levels of hormones within a conservative range is prudent. A daily dose of .625 mg of Premarin may result in a blood level of 100 picograms per milliliter (pg/mL) for one 57-year-old woman, yet may yield only 40 pg/mL for another woman of the same age. Since the Women's Health Initiative did not measure and record blood levels, we cannot know whether or not higher sustained blood levels of estrogen might have contributed to the small increased breast cancer risk that was reported.

Millions of women suffer menopausal symptoms, which

include "hot flashes," depression, headaches, mental fuzziness, memory impairment, fatigue, vaginal atrophy, and dryness— and the eventual risk of osteoporosis. Estrogen supplemental therapy is very helpful for many of these women, who now, more than ever, face a dilemma of choice.

We do know that:

- If we have a uterus, we need some progestin to protect it.
- Natural micronized progesterone, 200 mg for twelve days per month, will protect the uterus and interfere least with the beneficial effects of estrogen on our heart and blood vessels.
- We need to work with a doctor who measures our serum levels of estrogen and prescribes dosages to keep them within a conservative range (80–150 pg/mL).
- Regular breast exams and yearly mammograms are important to screen for breast cancer. On hormones or off, we are all at risk.
- An annual vaginal ultrasound examination can monitor the ovaries and may detect ovarian cancer.
- There are no "black and white answers." Whatever you might wish, no one knows for certain what is best for *you*.

Unfortunately, the Women's Health Initiative was not designed to provide the knowledge we need as to the long-term risks and benefits of a regimen of postmenopausal hormone supplemental therapy most likely to be safe: estradiol (with levels monitored and dosages adjusted individually) and natural micronized progesterone, taken only twelve days per month.

I know, firsthand, that symptoms of natural hormone imbalances and deficiencies can be miserable enough to tip the balance for women going through menopausal changes in favor of taking the risk associated with using responsibly regulated hormone supplementation for relief.

Treating women suffering menopausal symptoms of hormonal imbalance and willing to take the inevitably as-yet unknown long-term risks is one matter.

Tampering with the hormonal climate of healthy menstruating women, including teenage girls whose lives stretch ahead for decades, for the purpose of "menstrual suppression" is, in a word, reckless.

I began this chapter with the letter from that unhappy woman who was injected with Depo-Provera for birth control and menstrual suppression. That drug threw a chemical monkey wrench into the intricate mechanism of her pituitary-ovarian feedback loops, reducing estrogen and testosterone levels and causing loss of sexual interest and response.

A method of birth control that has been promoted substantially in Third World countries and is in growing use among some populations in the United States and in Europe, Depo-Provera had an unusual and inauspicious beginning. In the early 1960s, pregnant women who had had problems sustaining pregnancy were given the injection based on a theory that it would help them to keep their pregnancy to term. Here is the troubling story.

Chapter 5

Medical Experiments and My Father's Hat

●　　　●　　　●　　　●　　　●

Research in the medical archives can be something like an archaeological dig. Studying old published papers, some of which make reference to *unpublished* studies, can uncover layers of historical discoveries and allow a sobering look at the potential costs to human subjects of medical experimentation. From his book, *Is Menstruation Obsolete?* we learn that Dr. Elsimar Coutinho pioneered the development of Depo-Provera for contraceptive purposes. We also learn something about the story of the first clinical experiments with this drug that must, at the time, for a time, have been experienced as catastrophic for women desperately trying to have babies.

Early in his career, 1959, Dr. Coutinho was a "guest investigator" in the laboratory of Dr. George Corner at the Rockefeller Institute for Medical Research. Coutinho's early interest was the study of progesterone's natural functions in

maintaining pregnancy by preserving the integrity of the lining of the uterus and by suppressing uterine contractions.

In the 1950s, a synthetic progestin, medroxyprogesterone
acetate ("MPA"), was developed by Upjohn Pharmaceuticals.
(The term "progestin" applies to any formula that has
progesterone-like actions, including progesterone itself.) The
injectable form of MPA, in today's specific and approved
dosage, has become what we now know as Depo-Provera
(DMPA). By the early '60s, MPA was cleared by the Food and
Drug Administration for clinical trials to prevent late-term
spontaneous abortion and premature delivery.

With reasonably founded expectation that Depo-Provera
could help women successfully carry a pregnancy to full term,
Dr. Coutinho recruited women in Brazil with a history of
repeated spontaneous abortion or premature labor for an
experiment that would prove to give way to worry. Big time.

*The injected progestin failed to prevent abortion. What's worse,
it induced temporary sterility. In fact, some of the women hoping
to have a baby were sterile for a year and a half.*

The women whose pregnancies had failed did not begin to
ovulate. They did not menstruate. The injected hormone had
induced menstrual suppression. During the extended period of
menstrual suppression, no one could have known when, if
ever, these women would be able to conceive again.

*I could find no publication of this ill-fated experiment in the
medical literature.*

While distinctly unfortunate for the women who served as
test subjects, the experiment proved serendipitous for the

researchers, who subsequently ran a study and published a paper on the use of Depo-Provera as an innovative, injectable, long-acting contraceptive. I had no difficulty finding the 1966 paper reporting this followup experiment and groundbreaking news of "the use of an injected progestin *for the purpose of contraception.*" With Dr. Coutinho listed as lead author, this publication is entitled "Reversible Sterility Induced by Medroxy-progesterone Injections."

In the Introduction to *Is Menstruation Obsolete?* Dr. Coutinho describes his early (and apparently unpublished) experiment:

> *In our study, by the scheduled six-month followup visit after stopping Depo-Provera treatment, to our surprise, none of the women had resumed ovulating. Therefore, they had not menstruated during the half-year. Soon after the six-month check-up, however, the women started to ovulate and become pregnant again.*

A checkup sounds like a normal event, yet what was happening to these women was anything *but* normal.

Dr. Coutinho makes no mention of the misery that his study must have generated for the women and their partners and families. He says nothing about the worries and concerns that he and the other investigators surely must have had in response to the unforeseen developments. He does direct our attention to the fact that "the study serendipitously led to the discovery of the first long-acting injectable contraceptive."

To study and evaluate the information in Coutinho's book praising the benefits of menstrual suppression, I attempted to research the sources and bibliographic references cited. The task was confounded by the listings being run together in fine print, with no provision for discerning which reference was purported to support which fact. In my broad research I obtained, along with hundreds of papers by other investigators, all of the publications I could find on which Coutinho was listed as an author. I wanted to learn what I could about the scientific thinking and creative ideas of the doctor who suggests that menstruation is "obsolete."

I found in the archives a brief letter published in the *Lancet* of June 12, 1982, entitled "Kaposi's Sarcoma and the Use of Oestrogen By Male Homosexuals." Dr. Coutinho writes: *Although little is known of the prolonged effects of oestrogen [a spelling for "estrogen" used in the UK] on the immune response, its role in the depression of cell-mediated immunity has been well documented.* He goes on to say

> *Young male homosexuals take oestrogens for long periods to feminize their bodies and voices. This uncontrolled use of oestrogen by male homosexuals, although a common practice around the world, is especially prevalent in big cities, such as New York. Female homosexuals have no use for oestrogens or oral contraceptives and are, therefore, free from the immunosuppression which afflicts their male counterparts who attempt to change their appearances by hormonal treatment.*

The AIDS virus was soon to be identified as the agent wreaking havoc on the population suffering from Kaposi's sarcoma and other diseases that attack persons with weakened immune systems. Most of the AIDS sufferers, but not all of them, were male homosexuals.

Certainly, no clinician deserves censure for suggesting an approach, though it might later prove faulty, based on a balanced view of recognized phenomena and principles. However, any fair reading of Dr. Coutinho's letter finds it to raise questions about what appears to be irrational, if original, analysis.

He cites no source of empirical knowledge or scientific study to support the generalization that *young male homosexuals [especially those living in big cities, like New York] take oestrogens for long periods to feminize their bodies and voices.*

If Dr. Coutinho had suggested that, in the population of homosexual men, the potential connection between estrogen use and Kaposi's sarcoma might be a fruitful direction for scientific investigation, *that* would have framed the topic in a rational way. If he had wanted to make the point that women's bodies (*all* women's bodies—both heterosexual and homosexual) produce estrogen, but in levels more moderate than those achieved by extreme dosage of estrogen by *some* homosexual men, he would have made some sense. As it is, his pointed reference to homosexual women has no relevance to the unsupported point he makes about homosexual men. His suggestion that male homosexuals were at risk for immunosuppression "because they used estrogen" and that female homosexuals were not at risk "because they didn't" just does not make sense at all.

Reviewing the first published experiment of the use of injected MPA led me to reports of other experiments on other aspects of women's reproductive physiology, experiments conducted by investigators here in the United States that I found so disturbing that, for a time, I considered abandoning my research altogether. I didn't have the stomach for what I had to read. I chose to put aside those papers and to concentrate my attention on the remaining broad range of material essential to a responsible evaluation of the consequences of menstrual suppression.

Over a period of a year and a half, I located, reviewed, and

evaluated hundreds of relevant articles, nearly all of them generated by research carried out in more recent years. All the
while, that haunting stack of journal articles sat on the rug of
my office, sending a steady message. I had been so rattled by
their content that I resisted paying attention to what they were
telling me. Finally, as I sat down to write this book, I couldn't
avoid them any longer.

As a consequence, I have learned more than I want to
know of the troubling history of the lack of protection for
research subjects of clinical experiments on humans—and I am
not referring to the atrocities performed by doctors in the
concentration camps of Nazi Germany. Researchers in the
United States and elsewhere were not *required* to meet any set
of established ethical standards in experiments on women,
men, or children for nearly thirty years following the end of
World War II.

I was born in 1939. Television didn't come into my life
until I was ten, and "the movies" had a strong sensory impact.
Early on, I remember hiding my face behind my father's hat
when the MGM lion roared. The movies included cartoons
and newsreels, "Movietone News" and "Pathe News," with
footage of The War. Nothing effectively shielded me from see-
ing and hearing some of what was filmed at the concentration
camps—the horror of unspeakable violations. I was jolted by a
similar visceral response when I read publications of some of
the experiments performed on women here in the United
States in the 1960s and '70s—research that (as I subsequently
learned and was shocked to find) at the time met "the standards
of the day."

A helpful précis of the history of the first international
guidelines for the protection of human subjects of medical

research was published by the American Medical Association in
February 2001:

> *The Declaration of Helsinki emerged in the aftermath of World
> War II as one of the guidelines of biomedical ethical conduct. The
> Nuremberg Code (of 1948) had been formulated as a response
> to the judicial condemnation of the acts of Nazi physicians, and
> did not specifically address human subject research in the context
> of the patient-physician relationship.*
>
> *In 1964, the World Medical Association adopted the
> Helsinki Declaration as a response to concerns regarding research
> on patient populations. The primary purpose of the accord was to
> assert the interests of the individual patient before those of society.*

In reviewing the papers in that stack on the rug, the words
of the critical ethical mandate, "to assert the interests of the
individual patient before those of society," screamed out for
attention.

I have no doubt that society has benefited from some of the
information obtained through many of the studies in that collection, and through others like them. Neither have I doubt
that the interests of the individual patients in many of these
instances were violated. I cannot believe that any of the
research projects reported in the papers to which I refer meet
the standards of today, the standards enforced by the Office for
Human Research Protections (OHRP) of the United States
Department of Health and Human Services—an office that
thankfully has, at least today in the United States, a lot of clout.
It is painful to realize that that agency, those standards, and that
power were so long in coming.

The present-day protections were put into place by baby-steps. The first governmental agency involved, in 1962, was the United States Food and Drug Administration (FDA). The Kefauver-Harris Amendments made "informed consent" a requirement in human testing of drugs and cosmetics. Signed consent was not required.

Gradually the FDA policies were strengthened—but were limited in their power, since they applied only to studies of products regulated by the FDA. It appears that the studies at issue in my stack did not require FDA approval.

I learned from Dr. Michael Carome, director of the Division of Compliance Oversight at the Office for Human Research Protections, that it was not until the signing of the National Research Act in 1974 that the United States federal government established, as a part of the National Institutes for Health, the Office for Protection from Research Risk, which had the responsibility to oversee risks to human research subjects as well as matters pertaining to laboratory animal welfare.

In June 2000, the federal government established, as a separate and further-empowered agency of the United States Department of Health and Human Services, the Office for Human Research Protections. March 18, 2002, will go down in the history of biomedical ethics as the date that the authority of an agency of the United States government finally extended its protections of human research subjects to "international functions."

While the authority of OHRP is specific to experiments that are federally funded and does not technically extend to privately funded research, OHRP provides guidelines to private research institutions. In practical terms, on the basis of its economic and political authority and power, the scope of the powers of OHRP are not absolute, but are considerable. Institutions that don't want to risk losing grant money funded by agencies of the United States government had better meet OHRP standards for *all* the research they conduct.

There was no Office for Human Research Protections looking out for the women who participated in the experiments reported in that pile of papers on my office rug.

The 1964 Declaration of Helsinki is a document with ethical guidelines of wisdom and grace. A few of its basic principles:

- Concern for the interests of the subject must always prevail over the interest of science or society.
- Each potential subject must be adequately informed of the aims, methods, anticipated benefits, and potential hazards of the study and the discomfort it may entail.
- He or she should be informed that he or she is at liberty to abstain from participation in the study and that he or she is free to withdraw consent to participate at any time.
- The physician can combine medical research with professional care, the objective being the acquisition of new medical knowledge, only to the extent that medical research is justified by its potential diagnostic or therapeutic value for the patient.

The papers in my stack showed the treatment of the women in the studies they reported to fall seriously short of adherence to these principles.

In researching the history and current-day status of biomedical ethics, I contacted several experts—and left unanswered requests with several more. It is a busy field, these days. Like a hands-on CEO who answers his own telephone, Dr. Jonathan Moreno came right on the line. I couldn't believe my good fortune. Dr. Moreno is director for the Center for Biomedical Ethics at the University of Virginia Health System, has served as senior staff for two presidential commissions, and has been senior consultant to the National Bioethics Advisory.

When I revealed my findings in the medical literature to him, Dr. Moreno's first response was, "Well, you've got another book there." And my response was, "It's too dark for me." I don't have the stomach or the heart to be an investigative reporter on this subject. I'll stick to shedding light on the consequences of menstrual suppression.

For more than a year, since my first reading of those papers, the relevance of this darker material to the subject of "no periods" was not clear to me. Still, I couldn't shake the sense that there *was* an essential link. Finally, I knew. The history of exploitation of women as a vulnerable population for biomedical research has disturbing resonance with today's movement to sell women on the idea that menstruation is "obsolete." The women vulnerable to the trauma of those early experiments no doubt trusted that "the doctor knew best." Women today, even women living in "developed countries," are vulnerable to assurances that menstrual suppression is innocuous—that "the doctor knows best."

Women today remain vulnerable to the serious consequences of misplaced trust and exploitation.

I will provide, here, my father's hat for those who trust my judgment sufficiently to spare themselves the details. For any who want to look at the studies, I have provided a few of the citations in the chapter notes. Let me say, again, that **with respect to biomedical ethics, these studies met the standards of the day.** The painful truth is that a comprehensive review of the relevant published literature would reveal similar studies conducted by many other researchers all over the world. I am sure that books and articles on the history of medical ethics have addressed the subject. Nothing but more pain would be served by more detail.

Somewhere in my research for *The Hormone of Desire* I read a commentary that said that the use of hormone supplemental therapy for menopausal women is the largest uncontrolled experiment in medical science. In light of the "anti-period movement" afoot, I would amend that statement.

Manipulating women's reproductive hormonal chemistry for the purpose of menstrual suppression would be the largest uncontrolled experiment in the history of medical science. Hands down.

Twenty years ago, Dr. Coutinho had the idea that the epidemic of Kaposi's sarcoma was caused by homosexual men's use of estrogen. Today we all know better. Today Dr. Coutinho thinks that menstrual suppression is a good idea. It will be a long time before we all know for sure.

Chapter 6

The Truth About
"The Shot"

Depo-Provera, the drug that was developed to sustain pregnancy but whose effect was to produce temporary sterility and menstrual suppression, has been in use worldwide, as a contraceptive, since 1964. Today Depo-Provera is being injected into 2.5 million American women and 10 million women worldwide. While some are not unduly bothered by side effects, other women, like the woman whose letter we read in Chapter Four, suffer a range of miseries, including interference with sexual sensitivity and pleasure. One of the most serious undesirable effects of Depo-Provera, and one that women injected with it cannot feel and, if they are not told, cannot suspect, is to demineralize their bones, putting women, even teenage girls, at increased risk for osteoporosis.

Commonly referred to as "the shot," one injection of Depo-Provera every three months does the job of interfering with the normal maturation of eggs in the ovaries, of altering cervical mucus, and of suppressing the normal production of estrogen and testosterone.

Depo-Provera was tested (and obtained early approval for use) by poor women in underdeveloped countries. However, the shot was not approved for marketing in the United States until 1992. One issue that held up approval was the FDA's concern about the implications of early experiments that showed Depo-Provera to cause malignant mammary tumors (breast cancer) in beagles.

New Zealand was one "developed" country that gave early approval (1969) for the use of Depo-Provera. Twenty years of use there have provided researchers with data to evaluate breast cancer risk, and the conclusions of the study are not fully reassuring. The best that the investigators could do was to offer a vague statement: "These finding suggest that medroxyprogesterone may increase the risk of breast cancer in young women."

A 1995 analysis of the data collected by the World Health Organization pooled with that of the New Zealand researchers concluded that women considering the use of Depo-Provera "should be advised of the possibility that the drug might accelerate growth of occult [hidden] tumours [of the breast]." What this seems to mean is that the data did not reflect a clear and significant increased breast cancer risk with use of DMPA. If there were no other serious consequences to the use of this drug, the risk of breast cancer might not be a determining factor.

With regard to other cancer risks:

Two additional studies conducted by the World Health Organization have shown that the shot appears neither to increase nor to decrease the risks of ovarian or cervical cancer. DMPA does, like all progestins, have a definite protective effect on the lining of the uterus. However, there are safer and more moderate ways to use progestin to safeguard the endometrium from malignant change. I do not believe that the use of Depo-Provera, with its side effects and risks, is the progestin of choice for this purpose.

While concerns about heightened risk of breast cancer have earned a place on the sidelines, what *is* of very substantial concern, about which not enough noise has been made, is the fact that:

Depo-Provera causes bone loss.

Bone may seem as solid as stone, but it is not a static tissue. The physiology of bone growth and bone loss is exceedingly complex. By now you must know that when I say "complex," I mean *COMPLEX*. We build our bones and reabsorb minerals from them into our bloodstream continuously. I think we can manage without the details of the biochemistry.

Let's simply look at these facts:

- We have achieved our "peak bone density"—the strongest our bones will ever be—by the time we are twenty.
- Vital growth and strengthening of our bones occurs during our teenage years.
- Teenagers represent a large target population for the use of Depo-Provera.

To develop and to maintain healthy bones, girls and women need both enough calcium in their diet *and* high enough (normal) levels of estrogen and testosterone in their bodies. When Depo-Provera throws a hormonal monkey wrench into the workings of the normal menstrual cycle, it reduces the levels of estrogen and testosterone far below what's needed to help bones grow and to keep them strong.

A 1996 editorial in the *Journal of Clinical Endocrinology and Metabolism* emphasizes that normal bone growth and strengthening during puberty is critical for the health of bones over a lifetime. I was startled to read the extreme proposition of the "authority" on menstrual suppression, Dr. Elsimar Coutinho, who suggested that girls attempt to delay the onset of their first menstrual period by means of a regimen of superstrenuous exercise. Dr. Coutinho says, "Those who are willing to undertake the conscientious practice of exercise, whether sport or dance, before the first menstrual period, can delay the onset of the menarche for several years."

This is puzzling advice, since girls who exercise strenuously to the point of suppressing menstruation can be of concern to their knowledgeable doctors, who monitor bone density and, when appropriate, may encourage some moderation in exercise. Suppressing menstruation in pubertal or teenage girls can result in suppressing the normal levels of critical bone-building hormones, with potentially serious consequences in the form of increased risk of fractures and early development of osteoporosis—and with additionally detrimental effects on psychosexual development.

A profoundly important study measured intermittently over a two-year period the bone density of a group of normal adolescent girls who were not using any drug. They found that, over this period of time, the girls GAINED 9.5 percent in the density of their bones. Measurements of bone density of a similar group of adolescents who were being treated with Depo-Provera showed that this group suffered a LOSS of bone density of more than 3.1 percent, for an overall LOSS of bone density in the girls who had been injected with Depo-Provera of 12 percent. In the language of bone physiology, 12 percent is a lot of bone to lose—a seriously worrisome number. Warning of just this circumstance as a consequence of menstrual suppression, Dr. Winnifred Cutler, an authority on issues of women's health, has said:

"Young women develop old women's bones."

It's not just adolescents who are vulnerable to the bone-thinning effects of DMPA. Young women past their teenage years and older women who use Depo-Provera suffer serious bone loss as well. The population of women in New Zealand who have had access to the drug over the past forty years has been examined to learn its longer-term effects. The New Zealand studies and several others, including two carried out in the United States (Washington and Texas) confirm Depo-Provera's damaging effect on bones. The New Zealand researchers have put the matter very strongly:

"Use of DMPA (Depo-Provera) should be considered a potential risk factor for osteoporosis."

Labeling Depo-Provera "a risk factor for osteoporosis" is a serious indictment. The familiar list of risk factors until recently includes:

1. age (bone density diminishes normally with aging),
2. race (Caucasian and Asian women are more at risk),
3. history of inadequate dietary calcium,
4. smoking (not good for bones, either),

5. alcohol use (more than two drinks per day),
6. steroid medication (if used for any length of time).

Now, to this list we must add:

7. Depo-Provera (a serious risk if used as a teenager, or
for a "significant length of time" as an adult).

It turns out that a "significant length of time" could be a matter of *months,* not years. An article published in the *Journal of Reproductive Medicine* in 1999 and written by physicians at the army base in Tacoma, Washington, reported the case of a "33-year-old healthy, active woman" who lost 12.4 percent of her hip bone density and developed painful stress fractures in her legs "after receiving only three injections of Depo-Provera at ten-week intervals." That calculates out to twenty weeks from the date of the first injection until the diagnosis of the fractures. There was nothing in her medical history to account for this woman's particular susceptibility to rapid bone loss with her use of DMPA. This is another example of the range of women's complex physiology. We simply don't know enough to explain the constellation of differences in reaction to hormones and to drugs from woman to woman.

A foundational leitmotiv that I could include in each chapter:

Without an appreciation of the complexity of hormones' effects upon one another and of their far-reaching effects on every organ system in the body, we are not equipped to understand the risks of hormonal manipulation and disruption of the normal menstrual cycle.

With an appreciation of this complexity, we cannot be convinced that menstrual suppression is without harmful effects and future risk.

Too many physicians who offer to prescribe Depo-Provera for adolescent girls do not inform them or their parents about the risk to bones that this drug poses. Proponents of its use emphasize that the bone density loss "appears reversible following discontinuation of the drug." Such "reassurance" is irresponsible. Bone loss to teenagers does damage to bone that cannot be remedied *even with discontinuation of the drug.* I am troubled that proponents of Depo-Provera will not go so far as to advise AGAINST long-term use. Since each injection lasts three months, it is unclear just what "long term use" means. The longer a woman uses the drug, the more bone she will lose. Five months was long enough for the woman reported in the study we have cited to lose enough bone to develop stress fractures in her legs.

One other potentially serious consequence of Depo-Provera use is its undesirable effect on blood cholesterol.

A World Health Organization study measured the effects of Depo-Provera on women in Thailand, New Zealand, and Mexico who had been injected with the drug for periods of three to nine years. The authors concluded, "Long-term use of DMPA induces moderate changes in lipid metabolism which are unfavourable in terms of risk for atherosclerosis." They urged that "this should be borne in mind when weighing the overall risks and benefits of this contraceptive method for a potential user."

Are women who are advised to use Depo-Provera told about this risk?

A word about "side effects." I was taught in my pharmacology course in medical school that there really is no such entity! The fact is, *all* effects of a drug are, simply, its EFFECTS. We call some of them side effects when they are not the ones we are aiming for. With regard to its targeted effect, Depo-Provera IS a very effective contraceptive. The effects we would prefer it did not have include:

• Initial Bleeding and Spotting

The prospect of "no more periods" is what is promised to many women as a selling point for the injection. Most women spot and bleed intermittently following the first injection or two, but tend to develop oligomenorrhea (scant bleeding) or amenorrhea (no bleeding) after subsequent injections. Many women find the unpredictable vaginal bleeding troublesome enough to quit using the shot. One woman I spoke to told me that she bled nonstop for six months after starting on DMPA. One publication noted that some of the women who achieve complete menstrual suppression are unhappy about not having their periods "because they have no reassurance without vaginal bleeding that they are not pregnant." Some clinics that provide DMPA injections perform routine pregnancy tests before each subsequent shot to address this concern.

• Weight Gain

Every study evaluating the subject reported that women using Depo-Provera gained weight. Research shows that the increased appetite that troubles women using the shot may be due to a direct effect on the brain, where a particular set of neurons tends to accumulate concentrations of the drug. The amount of weight gain reported ranged widely depending on the population examined. A Milwaukee study showed that its population of African-American teenage girls gained twelve to eighteen pounds over a period of seventeen months. Another study of "73 teenage girls from a state-funded pregnancy prevention clinic and 60 girls from a private clinic" reported a weight gain range of from 8 to 10 pounds.

Just as we must face the reality that there are no easy answers to the problem of teenage pregnancy, we must acknowledge that Depo-Provera is neither a fully safe nor pleasant solution.

One study that described its experience with the use of Depo-Provera in adolescent girls appeared to be straining to put a good face on the data. Having made the point that "more than one million teen pregnancies in the United States each year create profound costs both to individuals and society," the author went on to report that 90 percent (of the girls who were injected with the drug) stated that they were "very happy" or "a little happy" with DMPA. To my way of thinking, "a little happy" is a far distance from "very happy"—quite a range of options to clump together in one statistic. It doesn't come as a surprise to learn that "in the same survey, 40 percent were unhappy with the side effects."

Adult women who use Depo-Provera gain weight, too, but to a less dramatic degree than the teenagers. A United States study reported that weight gain "was an important reason for stopping" (the injections). A New Zealand survey of women aged twenty-five to fifty-four also reported weight gain as a common reason for discontinuance.

• Sexual Side Effects

As we discussed in Chapter Four, Depo-Provera can wreak havoc on a woman's sexual libido and response. One paper reported that "overall, 56% [of the users] reported less interest in sex, and 55% reported less frequent sex." The subjects studied were teenage girls, and the author of this paper presented this figure as an apparently *positive* finding. By contrast, papers reporting libido changes in older women play down the importance of decreased libido as a side effect. Here is one case study that provides an impressive example of this bias:

> *"A 28-year-old married woman returns for her annual check-up after 1 year of DMPA. Overall, she is pleased but notes her sex drive has so declined it is beginning to affect her marriage."*

This sounds pretty serious to me. However, rather than discuss the advisability for this woman to stop the shot and use another method of birth control, the author of the paper comments:

> *"Libido is influenced by many factors, including a woman's relationship with her partner. Excluding marital problems, hormonal contraceptives can reduce ovarian production of testosterone, potentially reducing libido."*

(He's got that right!) He goes on:

> *"DMPA may decrease testosterone levels more than lower-dose hormonal methods."*

(YOU BET!) And he concludes:

> *"For ongoing DMPA users, consider low-dose combination estrogen/androgen supplementation (for example, Estratest H.S.)."*

EGAD. Speaking with reference to a woman who says that her sex drive is gone and that she and her marriage are suffering, he actually suggests that she *stay* on the shot and add some *more* hormones! To top it off, Estratest H.S. ("Half Strength") has *twice* the amount of testosterone most women need (and so is not "low dose" except in comparison with Estratest full strength, which has five times the dose of testosterone I most commonly recommend).

• Depression/Anxiety/"PMS"

I have discovered that, with all its drawbacks, the shot is being prescribed by some U.S. obstetricians in private practice, who recommend it for contraception to women after childbirth—a time when their bodies are making the transition back from the high hormone levels of pregnancy. I met a woman at an art show who had had the shot after the birth of her baby. When her doctor told her about one injection every three months—and no periods—it sounded pretty good to her. She had no way of knowing that, while she nursed her baby, building its bones with the calcium from her breast milk, her own bones were losing mineralization as a consequence of the drug that had been injected into her body. In terms of side effects, she was fortunate and tolerated the drug pretty well. Pretty well, that is, until she decided to allow her body to resume its normal hormonal cycling and to "stop having the shot." At that point, she said, she became horribly depressed.

This young woman was emphatic about how much she suffered, for several months, until the depression let up. When we spoke, she had not yet begun having normal periods. (If a woman stops using Depo-Provera and wants to get pregnant, the average time to return to fertility is ten months, with some women whose menstrual cycle does not return to normal for up to eighteen months.)

Reports of the depressive effects of Depo-Provera abound in the literature. One of the studies I read confirmed the common incidence of this anecdotal account, reporting "women who discontinued DMPA were 60% more likely to report depressive symptoms than non-DMPA–using women."

Here's a list with brief descriptions of the remaining cluster of more frequently seen side effects of Depo-Provera:

- **Headaches:** the most common side effect
- **Abdominal distress/pain/nausea/bloating/constipation:** Depo-Provera loosens the tone of the muscle in the gastrointestinal tract
- **Hot flashes, vaginal dryness, and other menopausal symptoms:** caused by the bottomed-out levels of estrogen and testosterone that also cause the loss of bone density we discussed at the start of this chapter

The one potentially beneficial consequence of the low estrogen state—a decreased risk of benign fibroid tumors of the uterus—is offset by the seriously increased risk to bone induced by Depo-Provera.

We have troubling evidence that many of the women who accept their doctors' recommendations to use DMPA are not only denied the information about prospective side effects, but also are treated dismissively when they return complaining of miserable problems caused by the drug. A website that has accumulated, in twelve months, 277 pages of letters from angry women suffering serious side effects of Depo-Provera was created by a woman worried about the consequences of her own miserable experience with the drug. The stories told by these women have disturbing common elements:

- Their doctors did not tell them what the side effects of the drug could be.
- Some doctors denied outright that the symptoms the women complained about could be caused by the Depo-Provera.

Here's a small sample of what these women have written:
A young woman from Canada:

> *I started taking Depo in Oct/2001 and then my last shot was Jan/2002—reason being—I gained 50 pounds during that time. Along with the weight gain, I had severe mood swings, absolutely no sex drive, dizzy spells, dry skin patches, headaches, anxiety attacks and lack of motivation.*
>
> **I feel like I am stuck in someone else's body.** *I used to be a healthy and active 25 year old. Now I just feel worn out and troubled, not to mention depressed.*
>
> **I feel like I was very misled by my doctor . . . the only thing she mentioned was the bonuses, like "no periods,"** *but I'd take the periods over feeling like I do today.*

A twenty-three-year-old woman from Maryland:

> *I have gained 40 pounds in six months, have the sex drive of an old woman (and the dryness of one too), I have aching joints and bleeding off and on for no reason, and I have such*

depression spells where all I want to do is die. I need to get this *@#$% out of my system. . . . **The doctors deny that any of*** ***this is caused by Depoprovera [sic], but strangely enough I*** ***did not have any of these problems before.***

A young woman in Newfoundland:

I have only been on the "shot" for two and a half months, *but already my body is going out of whack! I feel I want to* *jump out of my own skin. I am always sick, be it a headache,* *stomachache, or impossible fatigue. I feel I am getting worse* *every day.* ***I did not link these problems in any way with*** ***the Depo shot until I found this website.*** *I am now edu-* *cated thanks to you, and I will make sure that I will let every-* *one know just how dangerous this medication can be.*

A nineteen-year-old woman from the United States:

I have been taking the depo shot for two and a half years *now. I have experienced all of the side effects. I am very scared.* ***I had no idea that this could be what was making me feel*** ***so bad.***

These letters are from women who are suffering a range of undesirable side effects. Women who tolerate using DMPA without troubling side effects—and some women do—are at risk for bone thinning. Their doctors owe it to them to fore-warn them of this proven effect of the drug.

Women today remain vulnerable to the serious conse-quences of misplaced trust and exploitation.

I've interviewed a sampling of gynecologists for their opinions about Depo-Provera. Their responses reflected the populations of women in their practices. Doctors with middle- and upper-income women patients were the most outspoken in their negative attitudes. One said:

I NEVER give it. If a woman has a miserable reaction, you can't get it out. What are you going to do? If she feels rotten on the stuff, what are you going to do? You have to wait three months for it to wear off.

Another gynecologist was terse:

I think it should be taken off the market!

The sad truth is that for millions of women in a range of miserable circumstances across the world, Depo-Provera, with all its bone-thinning risks and potential for disturbing side effects, is a better choice than any other option they may have.

Women who *do* have an array of options and are told, "One shot every three months and NO PERIODS" must be given all the information we have, and we have plenty, to enable them to make their best choice.

Chapter 7

The More-or-Less Nonstop Birth Control Pill

No method of reversible birth control is more convenient, easy to use, and effective than the oral contraceptive pill. One hundred million women worldwide, including at least ten million American women, are on the Pill. Maybe you are one of them. If your circumstances of health and relationship meet the following criteria, the benefits may well exceed the risks for you to use the Pill for some period of your reproductive life:

- If you are a healthy woman;
- If you have no clotting disorders or relevant family history of clotting disorders; no liver problems; no high blood pressure or other cardiovascular disease;
- If you DO NOT SMOKE;
- If you are already sexually intimate exclusively with

ONE partner who is DEPENDABLY EXCLUSIVELY intimate with you;
and

- If your partner has NO SEXUALLY TRANSMIT-TED DISEASE, including the Humanpapilloma Virus,

Then you will have minimized (but not eliminated) the risks of using a carefully selected oral contraceptive. If your health and circumstances meet these criteria, the risks of extending the use of birth control pills for the purpose of menstrual suppression may not be much higher than using the Pill for contraception alone.

A second group of women whose risks/benefits can swing in favor of nonstop oral contraceptive use are women who suffer from debilitating illnesses that are exacerbated by the hormonal shifts of the menstrual cycle.

- Women who regularly experience severe migraine headaches in connection with their menstrual cycle *sometimes* have fewer headaches if they take birth control pills nonstop to keep the hormone milieu of their body stable. Some women's migraine headaches are made worse by the Pill—but that aggravation may be caused by the one-week withdrawal of hormones. Nonstop use might help some of these women.
- Women with a seizure disorder associated with the hormonal shifts of the menstrual cycle (an uncommon condition known as catamenial epilepsy) can sometimes benefit from nonstop use of oral contraceptives.
- Women with severe endometriosis, who bleed monthly not only from the uterus but also, painfully, into the

abdomen, are sometimes helped by nonstop use of
the Pill.

The most significant benefit of the birth control pill is its
use by women who are at particular risk of developing ovarian
cancer. Most studies have shown that the Pill can substantially
(up to 50 percent) reduce the risk of ovarian cancer. For these
women, nonstop oral contraceptive pill use is actually a "treatment of choice."

**For women who fit none of these sets of criteria, the risks over
the benefits of using the Pill are greater than you realize.**

The aim of this chapter is to lay out the particulars for you
to conduct your own risk/benefit evaluation, if you want to
make an informed decision about using "the more-or-less continuous birth control pill" for menstrual suppression.

In the 1960s, when it was first available, more than half of
all women using birth control were reported to be on the Pill.
Between 1973 and 1982, as it became apparent that women on
the Pill—even *young* women—were dying from heart attacks,
pulmonary embolism, and strokes, the use of the birth control
pill declined markedly. For a time following the introduction
of the "low dose" pills in the 1980s (developed with the expectation that they might prove to be "safer"), oral contraceptive
use leveled off for a time at 31 percent of all women using
contraceptives.

In 1988, with concerns about AIDS the focus of aggressive
media attention, oral contraceptive use began to drop further.
Use of the Pill leaves a woman fully at risk of infection with
sexually transmitted diseases. At the same time, and likely for

the same reasons, condom use has increased from 12 percent in 1982, to 15 percent in 1988, to 20 percent in 1995, the most recent year for which statistics were obtainable.

I was surprised to learn that "the most commonly reported method of contraception" reported in 1998 was "female sterilization." More than ten million (10.7 million) women of reproductive age in the United States have had their tubes tied. Still, as of that 1998 report, 10.4 million—or about 27 percent of American women practicing any form of birth control— used the Pill.

If you are taking oral contraceptives, perhaps you don't realize that your body is already being subjected to the hormonal effects of menstrual suppression. The "period" that you have after taking birth control pills for the usual twenty-one days **is not a menstrual period.** The usual twenty-eight-day birth control pill "cycle" **is not a menstrual cycle.**

Birth control pills work by shutting down the normal menstrual cycle.

"Sugar pills" or "blanks" contain no hormones. The vaginal bleeding that happens for most women in the fourth week of a birth control pill cycle occurs when the estrogen and progestin effects have been withdrawn, which causes the lining of the uterus to break down. That is why the "period" of bleeding for a woman on the Pill is known as "withdrawal bleeding" and not "menstruation."

The birth control pill "cycle" could originally have been established to be any length whatsoever. The twenty-eight-day-"cycle" regimen chosen by the original developers of the birth control pill created the *illusion* that the Pill was keeping physiological events normal. It is only an illusion. Nothing could be further from the truth.

Because the usual schedule of birth control pill use includes one week of sugar pills, women sometimes suffer symptoms (headaches, mood shifts) of hormone withdrawal. Researchers for the drug companies have been experimenting with a variety of hormone formulas and sequences, including some that add back hormones during the "blank" week, to try to address these problems.

Many of the pharmaceuticals that are presently being developed for menstrual suppression are birth control pills designed for more or less continuous use. One such drug will be packaged for ninety-one-day cycles, with eighty-four active pills followed by seven "sugar pills," which would allow for four "periods" a year. An MSNBC news feature: "Should monthly menstruation be optional?" (April 18, 2000) reported the pharmaceutical's inventor, Dr. Gary Hodges, to say:

There's no reason to think a cycle couldn't be even longer, but I chose ninety-one days for practical reasons—it works out to a nice, round four packs a year, and four periods a year may keep the amount of breakthrough bleeding down.

What Dr. Hodges means by "breakthrough bleeding" is that even on these pills that are designed to "do away with periods," women have irregular bleeding and spotting—more during the first several months, and varying in quantity from woman to woman. These variations are manifestations of women's normal hormonal complexity that fuels fundamental concern about the potential risks of menstrual suppression.

In that feature story about menstrual suppression, MSNBC

also quoted Dr. Gerson Weiss, chairman of the department of obstetrics and gynecology at New Jersey Medical School:

The side effects and complications of the pill will increase as more active pills are taken each year.

"Side effects and complications." What does he mean? Typical of the lack of balance in media coverage that hypes menstrual suppression, this vague, bland, and blanket statement is a pale counter to the excitement generated by advance promotion of pharmaceuticals to do away with the menstrual cycle that will be competing in a market currently valued at more than $2.2 billion annually.

"Side effects and complications." Here's what he means:

- Heart attacks,
- Strokes,
- Cancer of the cervix,
- Immune system compromise,
- Loss of sexual appetite and reduced sexual response,
- Depression.

Birth control pills throw a hormonal monkey wrench into the normal, intricate interplay of hormones and their effects not only on reproduction, but also on our blood vessels, our heart, our bones, our immune system, and our brain.

- Oral contraceptives stimulate the production of hormone binding globulins, which ties up our body's available testosterone.
- Reduced levels of available testosterone have negative

effects on sexual desire, sensitivity, and response, as well as on metabolism, muscle tone, mood, and cardiovascular health.

- The Pill reduces levels of ACTH, the pituitary hormone that stimulates the production of hormones from the adrenal cortex, including DHEAS (dehydroepiandrosterone-sulfate)—with damaging consequences to a woman's immune and stress responses.
- "Oral contraceptive users compared to nonusers showed lower NCA (natural cytotoxic activity)"—a protective immune response. Women using the Pill also demonstrated "an increased incidence of self-reported illness."
- "Oral contraceptive users may be at higher risk for certain stress-related disorders and are less well equipped to cope with times of prolonged physical or psychological stress."

"Side effects and complications!" JUST WHAT WOMEN NEED.

When, in my late twenties, I tried birth control pills for several months, I experienced a gradual decrease in any "monthly" withdrawal bleed, to the point where I didn't bleed at all. Aha! Menstrual suppression for sure. But I didn't like it. I just didn't feel normal. I missed my body's natural rhythms, the ebb and flow of energy, creativity, libido. At that time, I didn't know anything about "free" testosterone or sex hormone binding globulin. I just knew I didn't feel right. When I decided to stop taking oral contraceptives, I was relieved to get back to feeling like myself again. The convenience and ease of using the Pill had not been worth the sacrifice of my body's natural chemistry.

Dr. Elsimar Coutinho links his analysis of some women's unease with menstrual suppression and ignorance about their menstrual cycles—

Many women still view menstruation as a purifying mechanism that rids them of contaminated or bad blood.

—with what he clearly considers to be irrational:

Similarly, many women also associate menstruation with femininity, fertility, and youth, while considering the end of menstruation with aging and menopause.

What *is* menstruation, if it is not evidence of a woman's femininity and fertility? Proponents of menstrual suppression do not recognize and appreciate the richness of the full body/mind/spirit experience lived by a healthy, fertile-age woman.

As a consequence of the variety and complexity of hormonal tapestries from woman to woman, there is no one oral contraceptive formula that will dependably create even the illusion of a "normal" cycle for every woman. The same estrogen/progestin pharmaceutical that results in one woman's having three weeks without bleeding followed by several days of "withdrawal bleed" will cause another woman to have days throughout the month of spotting and bleeding, and another woman to have NO withdrawal bleed, even during a drug-free fourth week.

Birth control pill formulas whose proportion of estrogen to progestin is kept constant throughout the cycle (so-called monophasic oral contraceptives) are reported to result in less breakthrough bleeding than do formulas where the proportion of estrogen to progestin varies through the cycle (triphasic oral contraceptives). To reduce the incidence of bleeding and spotting, pharmaceuticals being developed for menstrual suppression are monophasic birth control pills.

Whether they are used in a monthly cycle or more continuously, there is a particular disadvantage to monophasic pills. Their steady stimulation of sex hormone binding globulin results in steady depression both of available testosterone, with resulting suppression of sexual interest and response, and of adrenal cortical hormones, with resulting reduced immune and stress response. The hormonal composition of the so-called triphasic pills varies a little from week to week, which allows for some flux in other hormone levels, and with a complex of effects from woman to woman.

Our leitmotiv belongs here:

Without an appreciation of the complexity of hormones' effects upon one another and of their far-reaching effects on every organ system in the body, we are not equipped to understand the risks of hormonal manipulation and disruption of the normal menstrual cycle.

With an appreciation of this complexity, we cannot be convinced that menstrual suppression is without harmful effects and future risk.

I have researched, studied, condensed, and highlighted a huge body of information published on the substantial cardiovascular risks to women on the Pill. If you don't want to read the information in detail, at least scan it for the bold type. It is important.

Cardiovascular Risks to Women Using Oral Contraceptive Pills

First, let's learn the language:

- "First generation pills" (introduced in the 1960s) contain very high doses (50 micrograms or more) of ethinyl estradiol and the progestins lynestrenol or norethisterone.
- "Second generation pills" (introduced in the early 1970s) contained lower doses (20 to 30 micrograms) of ethinyl estradiol and the progestin levonorgestrel.
- "Third generation pills" (introduced in the 1980s and 1990s) combined *the same lower doses of ethinyl estradiol as the "second generation pills,"* but with different progestins—desogestrel or gestodene.

During a woman's natural menstrual cycle, she benefits from a protective cyclical reduction in blood pressure—another built-in advantage of normal female physiology. Researchers have discovered something known as endothelin, a substance produced by the cells of the linings of blood vessels. Endothelin causes blood vessels to narrow, and, in this way, raises blood pressure. A woman whose normal menstrual cycle has not been tampered with has the benefit, for about half the month, of having lower levels of endothelin, and, consequently, lowered blood pressure. *Research has shown that this beneficial LOW-ERING of blood pressure is not present in women who take oral contraceptives.* It is not surprising that the Pill has been shown to raise a woman's blood pressure. Analysis of the data shows that:

Even small increases in blood pressure caused by oral contraceptives can account for major cardiovascular disease.

A worrying connection emerged in the years following the introduction of the birth control pill, where women who used first generation pills were discovered to be at increased risk of developing blood clots, pulmonary embolism, high blood pressure, heart attacks, and strokes. An impressive 1999 report in the *British Medical Journal* consisted of a twenty-five-year followup of forty-six thousand women who had used oral contraceptives. While some second generation pills were available in 1974, the women whose risks were reported in this study had used predominantly the lowest-dose first generation pills—containing 50 mg of estrogen.

These women were shown to have been about two and one half times more likely to die as a result of pulmonary embolism, heart attacks, and strokes than if they had never taken the Pill. The paper reported that "the excess mortality . . . fell with time." *This appears to be an encouraging statistic, but I couldn't help wondering whether the mortality figures improved with time because the women vulnerable to developing blood clots and to dying from heart attacks and strokes had either already died or been taken off the Pill.*

A 1981 publication in the *New England Journal of Medicine* opened with the following statement:

> **It is now established that in addition to increasing the risk of venous thromboembolic disease, oral contraceptives increase the risks of myocardial infarction, thrombotic stroke, and hemorrhagic stroke.**

What does this mean?

- "Myocardial infarction" means a heart attack—that heart muscle has been damaged as a result of a blood clot or arteriosclerotic narrowing/closing off in a coronary blood vessel (a blood vessel that supplies heart muscle itself).
- "Thrombotic stroke" happens when brain tissue has been damaged as the result of a clot blocking a blood vessel in the brain.
- "Hemorrhagic stroke" happens when brain tissue has been damaged as a result of a blood vessel in the brain that has burst. (High blood pressure can be one reason for hemorrhagic stroke.)

Birth control pills increase women's risks of all of these calamities.

Today's so-called low-dose oral contraceptives (second and third generation pills) were developed with the expectation that they would prove to be safer. Second generation pills somewhat reduced a woman's increased risk of heart attacks, but caused the levonorgestrel side effects of weight gain, acne, and adverse changes in blood cholesterol levels. Third generation pills were developed combining the same lowered dosage of potent estrogen with different progestins—partly to avoid the "levonorgestrel side effects."

The resulting effects on cardiovascular risks are neither simple nor reassuring. While the third generation pills have a significantly reduced heart attack risk, the risk of fatal pulmonary embolism has actually INCREASED.

Even more troubling, on February 7, 2002, a statement released from the meetings of the American Stroke Association (a division of the American Heart Association) reported:

*The risk of ischemic stroke in women using the "low dose"
pills (both second generation and third generation pills) was
actually HIGHER than that of today's smaller group of
women using the first generation pills.*

A rash of papers reports that third generation pills are associated with an even greater increased risk than ever of causing
clots to form in the deep veins of the legs and potentially to
travel to the lungs—a life-threatening condition known as pulmonary embolism. A statement describing the scope of the
problem was published in a 2002 paper:

*Because oral contraceptives are so widely used, they are respon-
sible for a large share, if not the majority, of all venous thromboses
in young women.*

In March 2002 Reuters Medical News reported a class
action trial on third-generation oral contraceptives in Britain,
a trial that follows "seven years of controversy over the safety
of the third-generation pill." The claimants "are believed to
include the families of five teenagers who died, as well as
young women who have been paralyzed and are now confined
to wheelchairs." The women bringing suit are claiming that
the drug manufacturers did not research the risks adequately
and provide warning of the true risks.

That Reuters report quoted a spokeswoman for the drug
manufacturer, who provided the following statistics, with
emphasis on the fact that they have been conveyed publicly in
the past and should qualify as adequate warning as to the risks
of these drugs:

Five of one hundred thousand women NOT taking oral contraceptives will develop a "thrombotic event" (deep vein clots, pulmonary embolism, heart attack, or stroke).

Fifteen of one hundred thousand women taking second-generation birth control pills will develop a "thrombotic event."

Twenty-five of one hundred thousand women taking third-generation birth control pills will develop a "thrombotic event."

A group of researchers at the European Institute of Health and Medical Sciences at the University of Surrey, U.K., has calculated that the true rate of "thrombotic events" is "probably nearer 37 per 100,000 exposed woman years." They calculate, in other words, that for every one hundred thousand women who use the newest (third generation) birth control pills for one year, thirty-seven women will develop blood clots and potential stroke. That figure is pretty disturbing to me. I think of the women in my city, consider one hundred thousand of them on birth control pills for a year, and imagine thirty-seven with dangerous blood clots and strokes. Teenagers. Young women. Mothers of children. Not a good thing.

Pharmaceutical representatives argue that the risk of developing blood clots is a threat for all women during pregnancy, and that the risk of the Pill is no greater. This line of argument is based on the assumption that if women didn't use oral contraceptives, they would get pregnant—and the fact that pregnancy carries its own increased risks of blood clots and stroke. But, of course, women do have a choice of other methods of contraception—methods that carry no increased risk of "thrombotic events."

Compounding the risk of blood clots, stroke, pulmonary

embolism, or heart attacks is the troubling number of women who smoke and are on the Pill. Doctors may recommend against oral contraceptives for women whose cardiovascular system is already compromised by high blood pressure or diabetes, but many physicians prescribe them for women who want them and are smokers.

Women who smoke and use birth control pills—even YOUNG women—are at substantially increased risk of blood clots and stroke.

Truly alarming is the fact that a quarter of all women who take oral contraceptives smoke—and of these, more than half smoke heavily (more than fifteen cigarettes per day). A paper published in the *American Journal of Obstetrics and Gynecology* in 1999 describes the problem of women smokers' use of oral contraceptives as "an urgent public health issue that may affect millions of American women."

Discouraging statistics released in October 2001 by the Centers for Disease Control and Prevention showed that there has been essentially no change in the number of smokers, a number "holding steady" at roughly one in four American adults. We can do the math. At least ten million American women use birth control pills; one in four are smokers. The urgent public health issue DOES affect millions of American women.

About one hundred million women worldwide use birth control pills. Tens of millions of women worldwide are at increased risk of cardiovascular death.

A consensus of the conference of the Association of Reproductive Health Professionals that was convened in 1999 to discuss the issue of risk to women smokers of using oral

contraceptives advised the following to physicians who prescribe oral contraceptives:

- All patients should be discouraged from smoking.

As though smokers don't know . . .

- Heavy smokers older than age thirty-five should not
  use oral contraceptives because of possible increased
  risk of cardiovascular disease.

This *is* a remarkably clear injunction.

- All smokers below age thirty-five may be advised to
  use the lowest available dose of oral contraceptive.

This one is hard to understand, since publications had been
reporting since 1995 that even the "low dose" pills carry substantial cardiovascular risk, and the third generation pills put
women at highest risk for clotting and its dangerous consequences.

**If the possibility of doing away with one's period
through the use of the more or less nonstop birth control pill is presented as innocuous, more women will use
oral contraceptives—many of them smokers—and more
women will die.**

A letter from a concerned British physician published in
the *Lancet* in August 1997 put the matter eloquently:

> *Although the incidence of fatal thromboembolism is
> small, we are dealing with a group of otherwise healthy*

*young women with what would otherwise be a long life
expectancy. . . . It is my firm belief that consideration
should be given to the idea that all prescribing doctors of
the combined oral contraceptive pill should possess a cer-
tificate of competency.*

Since no oral contraceptive pill is free of cardiovascular
risk, doctors who prescribe the Pill can do so responsibly
only by evaluating each woman's individual risk factors, to
try to determine whether she is more vulnerable to clotting
disorders, elevated blood pressure, or heart attacks. Some
choice, eh?

Recent research has shown that women with a particular
genetic makeup—women who carry a gene called factor V
Leiden—are at an even *higher* risk of having a "thrombotic
event" than others who use oral contraceptives. Out of a group
of women with no family history of clotting disorder who
developed clots while taking the Pill, 8 percent had the factor
V Leiden gene. Third generation oral contraceptives are certainly NOT the drugs of choice for these women. But how
can a woman know if she is genetically vulnerable? Genetic
testing is unheard of as a screening procedure for determining
the safest oral contraceptive for a particular woman. And how
many doctors have the knowledge and take the time to make
careful evaluations that minimize cardiovascular risk to women
choosing oral contraceptives?

So far, we've focused on the risks of the Pill to each indi-
vidual woman. The bigger picture carries bigger concerns.
Oral contraceptive use has contributed to the spread of a
potentially lethal sexually transmitted disease, ***in addition to the
AIDS virus,*** that has changed the health climate for everyone.
We are now faced with the epidemic spread of high-

risk strains of the Humanpapilloma Virus, the first virus known to cause cancer in solid tissue.

There is evidence to suggest that birth control pills may be more than a passive partner to this virus in causing cancer of the cervix, the risk of which is plaguing vulnerable women and worrying parents of teenage girls who are turning up with abnormal Pap smears. Here is what we all need to know.

Chapter 8

"The Pill" and the Virus That Causes Cancer

●　　　●　　　●　　　●　　　●

When I set out to do the research into the medical risks of menstrual suppression, I had no way of knowing that I would spend considerable time researching the role of oral contraceptives as a partner to a virus that causes cancer. I did know something about the Humanpapilloma Virus—commonly referred to as HPV. For some time, information had been making its way into public awareness about the association between HPV and cancer of the cervix (the opening of the uterus that extends into the vagina). A few years back I had read an article in the *New Yorker* by Dr. Jerome Groopman (the issue of September 13, 1999) that carried this alarming subtitle: ***"A Sometimes Lethal Sexual Epidemic That Condoms Can't Stop."***

Just at that time, one of the "twenty-something" patients in my psychiatric practice had turned up with abnormal Pap smears and had been diagnosed with HPV infection. She had been undergoing repeated specialized examinations of the tissue of her cervix, with biopsies of tissue that didn't look normal. Colposcopy was what that procedure was called. She hated it. I was worried about her.

One of the cases Dr. Groopman described was a young married woman he had treated who contributed to the statistic of the six thousand or so American women who die each year from cervical cancer. My research into the subject turned up the fact that at least 70 percent of HPV infections clear up on their own—that a woman's immune system can fight off the infection, and her Pap smears will revert to "normal." Thankfully, my patient was to be among this majority.

Near the beginning of my research into the risks of stopping periods through more or less continuous use of oral contraceptives, I found a 1999 *British Medical Journal* article reporting the results of a forward-looking study that had begun in 1968. The investigators followed the health profiles and causes of the deaths that had occurred in a large population of women (23,000) who were using oral contraceptives and those of a similar number of women who had never used them. The paper represented a "25 year follow up of a cohort of 46,000 women"—a very substantial collection of data.

When I reviewed the table of statistics that reported the "relative risk of death in users of oral contraceptives compared with 'never users,'" I found confirmation of what I already knew about the Pill's significant protective effect against ovarian cancer. The data also confirmed, clearly, the increased risk to women using oral contraceptives of dying from cardiovascular diseases. What WAS news to me was the alarming number of women who used the Pill and had died from cancer of the cervix. That risk appeared to increase over time. The longer that women used oral contraceptives, the more of them died of cervical cancer compared with women who had never used the Pill.

These statistics reinforced what had been reported in an earlier U.K. study, published in 1983, whose authors collected data about 6,838 women who were taking oral contraceptives, and compared this group's incidence of cervical cancer with that of a group of 3,154 women who were using the IUD. The study found that *all of the cases of invasive cervical cancer that were found occurred in the group of women using the Pill.* The authors concluded that "long-term users of oral contraceptives should have regular cervical cytological examinations (Pap smears)."

While I was gathering this information that linked oral contraceptive use with increased risk of cervical cancer, studies were turning up that implicated infection with the Humanpapilloma Virus as a cause of this same cancer. Initially, my thinking went something like this:

1. Women using oral contraceptives are at higher risk for cervical cancer.
2. Women using oral contraceptives have no protection from sexually transmitted diseases.
3. HPV is a sexually transmitted disease.
4. Infection with HPV causes cervical cancer.

The obvious conclusion seemed to be that women on the Pill were sitting ducks for HPV infection, which increased their risk for cervical cancer.

However, there were problems with this reasoning. For one, the U.K. study I have mentioned had compared data collected from two groups of women: one group using oral contraceptives and the other group *using the IUD*. **None of the women in either group was using a "barrier" method of birth control.** *Both groups were equivalently vulnerable to infection with sexually transmitted diseases.* We could say that BOTH groups were sitting ducks for HPV infection, yet only the women using oral contraceptives had developed cancer of the cervix.

There's another flaw in my simplistic reasoning:

We are ALL sitting ducks for HPV infection.

The only way to prevent infection with the Human-papilloma Virus is to avoid intimate contact—even skin-to-skin contact—with another infected person. The virus is very highly contagious and can be transmitted from the skin of the scrotum or even the thigh from one person to another, where it can spread, in women, to internal sexual organs, including the cervix. While condoms offer some protection against other sexually transmitted diseases, including the AIDS virus, *the only safe partnered sex is sex with a person who does not have a sexually transmittable disease.*

When I found a number of papers describing the joint contribution of oral contraceptives together with the Humanpapilloma Virus to the development of cervical cancer, I knew I was on to something important. The connections are there, and they are worrisome.

The first paper was a 1986 publication of a National Cancer Institute study that reported data collected from five geographic regions of the United States. At that time, HPV had not yet been identified as the cause of 99.7 percent of all cervical cancers. The investigators of the 1986 study named oral contraceptives as a risk factor for invasive cervical cancer, and went so far as to implicate the Pill as a potential **"co-carcinogen"** (a partner in causing cancer) with other potential risk factors, including HPV. They concluded that

> *oral contraceptives might influence cervical cancer risk by acting as promoters for other risk factors, including smoking and herpes-virus or papillomavirus infections.*

Between 1985 and 2001, the pieces of the puzzle gradually emerged and came together. By 1991, investigators were reporting that infection with the Humanpapilloma Virus was "a high risk factor" for cancer of the cervix. Today, HPV has been confirmed as the cause of 99.7 percent of all cervical cancers. The medical community knows and accepts the fact that "high risk strains" of HPV are the cause of virtually all cervical cancer. Pharmaceutical companies are busily working to develop vaccines against the high-risk strains of HPV. The FDA has recently given its approval for a screening test for diagnosing HPV using the same sample of tissue obtained for routine Pap testing.

The likelihood that oral contraceptives make women's tissues more susceptible to the cancer-causing effects of HPV is, at this point, very little publicized. The most "in your face" study, reported in March 2001 by a group of investigators from the University of Washington School of Medicine in Seattle, was entitled

> *Human Papillomavirus and Long-term Oral Contraceptive Use Increase the Risk of Adenocarcinoma "In Situ" [localized] of the Cervix.*

Examining the data of the past forty years, the authors found that *coinciding with the availability of oral contraceptives (in the 1960s) there is an increased incidence of cervical cancer.* They concluded, in precise and careful language, that the data supports a role for oral contraceptives *as a promoter of HPV-related (cervical) cancer development.*

Until I dug up the papers, I knew nothing about the Pill's contribution to cervical cancer. It took about ten years for the information about HPV to become mainstream. Ten more years of ignorance could cost too much.

Women today remain vulnerable to the serious consequences of misplaced trust and exploitation.

Women who are being encouraged NOW to use oral contraceptives more or less nonstop for the purpose of menstrual suppression must be aware of the growing body of evidence that:

Oral contraceptives decrease the likelihood that a woman who contracts Humanpapilloma Virus infection will fight it off.

Women who use oral contraceptives, whether on a monthly schedule or more or less nonstop for menstrual suppression, are at increased risk of developing cancer of the cervix.

Oral contraceptives have been in use for almost forty years. Within a few years of their first use, it became apparent that women on the Pill were dying—even some very young women—of heart attacks and strokes. Other medical consequences have taken longer to be recognized. We have convincing evidence, now, that the longer women remain on the

Pill, the higher their likelihood of developing cancer of the cervix. In terms of further increased risk, who knows *what* more or less nonstop use of the Pill for the purpose of menstrual suppression will generate?

Young women with cancerous changes on their cervix who must undergo repeated colposcopy and painful removal of lesions develop scarring that can interfere with fertility and cause complications with pregnancy and delivery. Although cervical cancer "can be cured" . . . it isn't always. Ask Dr. Groopman.

No way can I be convinced that menstrual suppression achieved by more or less nonstop use of the birth control pill is innocuous.

No way.

Chapter 9

The Sexiest Thing
About a Woman

Since March 1999, women from all parts of the world have been writing letters in response to the question posted on a website: "Would you stop menstruating, if you could?" Many women wrote yes to the prospect of an end to monthly cycling and bleeding, with all its "mess and discomfort." However, even without specific knowledge about the medical risks of menstrual suppression, a substantial number of the hundreds of women who responded wrote impressively intelligent, creative, and impassioned letters to say NO to the opportunity to stop their menstrual cycles.

This book is heavily weighted with scientific information about the medical risks of menstrual suppression. To round out the issue, I present a sampling of the other costs of menstrual suppression in the words of the women who are not willing to pay the price—and from one man who had something he wanted to say.

A woman from the United States:

> *I really can't believe that women could be so hateful to their own bodies! . . .*
>
> *What if someone actually said that menstrual cycles could be FUN, BEAUTIFUL, HEALTHY, MAGICAL? What if a whole generation of women were raised to believe that their periods were . . . good?*
>
> *I won't even bother arguing weather [sic] skipping periods is a health risk or not. But it should be obvious to anyone that self-loathing (especially about fundamental body functions) is definitely a health threat. I beg anyone who is complaining about her period to reconsider how they view their body. Your body does NOT have to be dirty, stinky, painful, troublesome, expensive, or controlled by artificial drugs. I have no interest arguing that our cycles make us "real women" either. I think the only issue of concern here is women who are INSULTING their own bodies. No negative attitude like that could make anything enjoyable. And no drug can cure a negative attitude like that.*

From a thirty-three-year-old woman:

> *I am taking a college class at the University of _____ called The Psychobiology of Women. The things I have learned about my body are amazing! It is like a symphony constantly playing, hormones from one are cueing another instrument to play. I feel that knowledge is the best key; once you understand what and why, it is much easier to handle once a month. I have so much more respect for MY symphony!*

A twenty-six-year-old American woman:

> *No, I don't think that I would get rid of my period if I could. For me, cramps are minor and isolated to the first few days of menstruation. I enjoy the cramps I get the same way I enjoy the muscle pain after a really good beneficial workout. I don't know why, but I feel sexy when I'm menstruating. I realized at some point in college that that was when I was most likely to get dolled up and go to parties. I think I met several boyfriends while menstruating. From ovulation through menstruation I am most interested in sex, most emotional, and also most able to achieve sexual climax. I think all of that is certainly worth a mess.*

A young teenage girl:

> *My mom told me the argument that menstruation is obsolete, and I was immediately disturbed. How much can science make us unnatural before we take responsibility for our actions instead of curbing our natural processes with modern "medicine"? There have to be some major changes in the body in such a drastic thing such as taking menstruation away for a period of months.*

From a Canadian woman:

> *My period is a source of power. It cycles with the moon, which is a symbol of power of women. I am in rhythm with the earth and other women in the world when I cycle. I find it amazing to feel my body ovulate, and then wait for the bleeding. I am a complex being because of the cycle and am thus*

capable of bringing forth life. I would NEVER choose to stop menstruating as it is a ritual that I value deeply.

I think the recent articles about the obsoleteness of menstruation are just another form of period shame that the media is trying to instill in women so that they can become the consumers of yet another unhealthy hazardous product that someone without a uterus invented.

A fourteen-year-old girl:

I am 14 and got my first period when I was 11. Would I stop menstruation if I could? No way! Our moontime is when our personal feminine magic is at its peak! Why would I want to give that up? Also, I'd never go on the pill. The periods you get on them aren't real. They're not your body's natural cycle, they're just when you take the sugar pills. I used to not like my period, but as soon as I got rid of that ridiculous Western view of menstruation being a nuisance and embraced it as a wonderful magical thing, my cramps and other symptoms dropped drastically.

A teenage student from Brazil:

I am a 16-year-old Brazilian student and I wouldn't stop menstruating even if one paid me. I started my periods when I was 11 and they are about five to six days long and are not very heavy, but I have some cramps in the first and second days. Right after I got my first period I went through a denial stage (I actually didn't like it back then), but nowadays I just love it.

I especially came to give menstruation its worth when I went on a diet and got very skinny, almost anorectic. I went for six straight months without menstruating and was getting really concerned. I read about it and realized something was wrong with me. That was the wake-up call I needed to get off that psycho's diet before I got really ill. I still can remember how relieving and delightful it was for me when I went to the bathroom and there it was: bloody underwear. I thought, "Now my body is functioning well, I am healthy."

I am a feminist and I don't intend to have children. Still, I'd rather menstruate than anything else in the world. That's a characteristic of my female body and a natural function, like urinating or evacuating. Heaven knows what side effects this Pill would have on me? How am I going to know if I am okay or not? However, I think if a woman is suffering and her period is a total disaster she should be able to go on without menstruating and having a normal life. This is a right every female in the world should have.

But I am proud of being a woman, therefore I am proud of menstruating! Sometimes only you know how much peace of mind a period can bring you. And you also learn a lot about you with your period. So, if you can, enjoy it!

A twenty-five-year-old woman:

I cannot believe how many women would stop if they had the chance, no questions asked. It is mind-boggling. Too many of these women have been taught to hate their bodies; it is so sad. Menstruation is NOT smelly or dirty or bad. I wouldn't stop if someone paid me.

One, we have cycles for a reason—just like other creatures—and we cannot know what the consequences would be, regardless of what these scientists would have you believe. Two, it reminds me that I am a woman and makes me feel feminine and powerful.

I've had my period since I was 11 years old. I am now 25 and looking forward to having my first child. I love my body and the power that resides within.

A young girl:

I am only 15 but I love my period. It is quite amazing that I can bleed profusely without perishing. My period makes me strong. My period tells me about my health. The internal clock I possess is disrupted in the case of tumor, stress, or vitamin deficiencies. Bleeding keeps me informed. Someday my period will tell me that I am pregnant. This is a secret that I will know first, before anyone else. Just me and my body will know. My period gives me power. I know the day and the hour of when it will come and it only hurts a little for a day.

An archaeology student from Chile:

I wouldn't stop menstruating if I could. I'm 20 years old and I've been having my periods since I was 11. When I was younger I would have said yes, but now I feel I'm used to it, I've accepted it as part of my life. To be completely honest, I don't think it's sacred, neither does it make me feel like a woman. To me it's just another body function. I don't like going to the bathroom either, but I won't stop going because I don't like it.

A thirty-year-old woman:

Stop menstruating: NEVER EVER EVER!
I understand it can suck, and it is messy, expensive and can be quite uncomfortable. But come on, women, it's what makes

us stand apart from the men. Our bodies have been designed this way during the course of hundreds of thousands of years for specific reasons and to mess with Mother Nature is inviting trouble. Instead of bowing to the men and buying in to their flimsy excuses of why women should stop menstruating, stand tall and proud because menstruating is what makes us the life bearers that we are. To agree with the men that we should take a pill to stop this powerful gift is the same as defecting to the other side. [I'm] 30, female and lovin' it!

A thirty-six-year-old American woman:

No way. My body will do it when it is good and ready, I trust my body to do what it needs. I find it absolutely terrifying that womyn [sic] would want to take some drug—such as Depo-Provera—to stop their periods. Stopping our periods can only have serious repercussions. I live in the United States and, unfortunately, the media has really turned females against their natural cycles.

A mother of four:

Stop my periods? NEVER!!! As cheesy as it sounds, it is a thing primeval. I love the vitality and the power I feel during my period, even when I'm tired. It separates us from the rest, we are alive and tapped in to each other when we menstruate. I have given birth to four children, and I consider menstruating a powerful, positive event, cleansing and wonderful.

I am not a hippie, or a New-Age touchy feely, just a 36-year-old woman, grateful that there are some things that men can't take away from us. This whole cessation of menstruation is a male fantasy. Men have tried for centuries to control us repro-

ductively, and this is one thing they can't have. Don't kid your-
selves, girls, if it's all about making menstruation convenient and
not messy for men—I say, Step aside, boys, and let the real men
through, ones that honor and respect our bodies for the powerful,
life-affirming machines that they are. Stop menstruating? What
next? Will we go back to chastity belts and burning women at
the stake? Give me a break!

From a thirty-two-year-old homeopathy student:

Haven't we all lost touch with our bodies and our selves!
Do we really think that we can bend and shape nature to suit
US and not pay a price for it? How arrogant we are. There is
not an allopathic drug that comes without side effects.

I wouldn't part with my periods for anything. And I believe
that the reason I do not suffer with them is because I appreciate
them and have never been taught to hate my body's natural
cycles.

I'm a homeopathic student and would strongly urge anyone
suffering with their periods to consider homeopathy as a real
alternative to conventional drugs—the results are amazing and
there is no fear of side effects!

A twenty-six-year-old Californian:

Stop my periods? No way—No how!!!
Menstruation is a wonderful part of being a woman, yeah
i[t']s uncomfortable and even painful but if you listen to your
body and react accordingly, it all falls into place!

As soon as I learned to love my body, myself and the fact
that I was/am a woman, menstruation was no longer a horrible
part of my life nor a time of dread. Loving me means loving

that time of the month for all its good and bad aspects. I know
this attitude makes me sound like a stereotypical "New Age
Northern Californian," but I can't begin to tell you how much
a positive attitude toward my menses and my body image has
changed my experiences menstruating. Don't stop menstruating,
it happens for a reason! It's not a disease, it's a state of
wellness.

A senior in college:

> *I am a 22-year-old in my last year at the University of*
> *_____, and I would NEVER surrender my right as a*
> *woman to menstruate. It is a miracle and a gift, and every*
> *month I rejoice in its arrival. It is a right of passage and a*
> *blessing bestowed on only half of the world. It enables us to*
> *give life. LIFE. To create, shelter, and give birth to another*
> *life—AMAZING. During my sister's pregnancy, labor and*
> *birth of my nephew, I was constantly amazed and often brought*
> *to tears. She and my nephew are a constant reminder of the*
> *power we have in our bleeding as a woman. I would never stop*
> *it. It would destroy all that is me. I am not a man, and I have*
> *never wished to be, but wishing for menstruation to cease would*
> *be like denying Mother Nature and convincing ourselves that*
> *we have the knowledge and wisdom to take over her job with*
> *drugs and pills.*
>
> *Live and let bleed;)*

And, from a man:

> *Menstruation is the sexiest thing about a woman; it also*
> *gives new life on this planet.*

Afterword

A child of five when we dropped The Bomb on Hiroshima and Nagasaki, a grade-school kid crouching under my desk during "duck and cover" drills, a tenth-grade biology student horrified to learn the costs to life on this planet of the detonation of nuclear weapons or of potential leaking of radiation from other nuclear devices-gone-wrong, I was a commencement speaker at Worcester's Classical High School on June 13, 1957.

I hadn't thought about that graduation day talk of long ago for decades and decades—until June 2002, when I was winding up the writing of this book. After the pleasure of composing the acknowledgments and the dedication, I invoked of my muse direction to a quotation of apt wisdom as an introduction to the core theme of the book. Nothing came.

A friend suggested I might find something useful in

Frankenstein—not the Mel Brooks movie, but the great novel written in 1818 by Mary Wollstonecraft Godwin Shelley. Not until I stood in the stacks at the Newton Public Library, browsing through their several editions of that novel, did I remember my childhood commencement address.

In 1957, the title of my talk was "*Frankenstein:* Mary Wollstonecraft Godwin Shelley."

At that time, I earnestly and simplistically drew on the aspect of her novel that illustrates the disaster of tampering with the natural order. I spoke of worries about the possibility of nuclear devastation and the risks to us all of messing with Mother Nature. I could not understand how the grown-ups of the world would, for *any* reason, make use of instruments of such potentially destructive power.

Here I am today, one of the grown-ups, educated and experienced in the specialty of women's health, and again focused on the hazards of tampering with the natural order.

Mary Shelley's book did not, this time, prove aptly quotable. I looked further and discovered, remarkably, that her mother, Mary Wollstonecraft, had authored the first great feminist treatise. Published in 1792, *A Vindication of the Rights of Woman* includes an extraordinarily fine analysis and exposition of the immorality of consigning women to lives of ignorance and trust. It was in this collection of essays that I found the line that belongs at the beginning of this book and is, as well, a thematic through-line in what I have written:

Without knowledge there can be no morality!

When first I read about the "anti-period movement," I already had enough knowledge of women's physiology to know that menstrual suppression was not without risk. Today, having researched and studied what there is to be known about the medical hazards of stopping women's menstrual cycles, I have more concerns than ever.

Knowledge is power.

May this book serve as an instrument of power in protecting and promoting women's health—for ourselves, for our daughters, for our granddaughters, and for their posterity.

S.R.
Newton, Massachusetts

Notes

Foreword

p.19 "The *New Yorker*": M. Gladwell, 2000 (first listing).

p.19 *"The Tipping Point":* M. Gladwell, 2000 (second listing).

p.20 "Dr. Jerome Sullivan's 'iron hypothesis'": J. L. Sullivan, 1981.

p.21 *"The Hormone of Desire":* S. Rako, 1999.

p.22 "That testosterone is essential for women's health": G. A. Bachman, 1999; E. Barrett-Connor, 1998; S. Davis, 1999; D. A. Metzger, 1998.

1. No More Periods?

p.27 "Since my research and teaching": S. Rako, 1996.

p.27 "This problem of potential bias": F. Davidoff, 2001 (all listings).

p.30 "The title of a book by Brazilian gynecologist": E. M. Coutinho, 1999.

2. The Blessings of the Curse

p.35 "I am prepared for the possibility": S. Rako, 1999.

p.36 "Dr. Semrad's wisdom": S. Rako, 1980.

p.39 "In 1959, biologists first described": P. Karlson, 1959.

p.40 "a fellow Wellesley alumna": M. K. McClintock, 1971.

p.40 "In 1980, researchers discovered": M. Russell, 1980.

p.40 "Between 1975 and 1986": W. B. Cutler (all references); N. McCoy, 1985.

p.40 "A group of Swiss researchers": C. Wedekind, 1995.

p.41 "a woman's preference for a male": C. Wedekind, 1995, 1997.

p.42 "A hot-off-the-press publication": S. Jacob, 2002.

p.42 "An article in *New Science* magazine": A. Motluk, 2001.

p.42 "Optimal MHC compatibility dramatically improves": C. Ober, 1983, 1987, 1992 (both listings).

3. The Iron Hypothesis

p.45 "More than twenty years ago, in the *Lancet*": J. L. Sullivan, 1981 (first listing).

p.46 "Imagine this poster material for blood donation drives": T. P. Tuomainen, 1997.

p.46 "Recommended dietary iron": USDA Nutrient Data Base for Standard Reference, Release 12, 1998.

p.47 "In 1989, the *American Heart Journal* published": J. L. Sullivan, 1989.

p.48 "In 1996, the *Journal of Clinical Epidemiology*": J. L. Sullivan, 1996.

p.49 "By 1998, Dr. Sullivan was not a lone voice": S. Kiechl, 1997; T. P. Tuomainen, 1998.

p.49 "In 1999, an impressive review": B. de Valk, 1999.

p.50 "In 2000, authors of an article": S. Penckofer, 2000.

p.51 "of all foods, *prunes* rank highest": USDA Nutrient Data Base for Standard Reference, Release 12, 1998.

p.52 "women who consumed 3,000 micrograms of Vitamin A": D. Feskanich, 2002; S. J. Whiting, 1999.

p.52 "Dr. Elsimar Coutinho is dismissive of": E. M. Coutinho, 1999.

4. The Blind Men and the Elephant

p.55 *"The Hormone of Desire":* S. Rako, 1999.

p.58 "It is the drug promoted by Dr. Elsimar Coutinho": E. M. Coutinho, 1999.

p.58 "As I describe in *The Hormone of Desire*": S. Rako, 1999.

p.59 "An endocrinologist's bible": S. S. C. Yen, 1991.

p.60 ***"the estrogen content even of 'low dose' oral contraceptives"***: A. A. Murphy, 1990; J. Bancroft, 1991.

p.63 "The Scharrers were husband and wife pioneering researchers": B. Scharrer, 1944, 1963.

p.64 "Let me quote a section from one of the more lucid texts": L. Speroff, 1999 (pages 43–44).

p.67 "In fact, estrogen can legitimately be considered": E. L. Klaiber, 1997; E. C. G. Grant, 1968.

p.68 "are instead prescribed an SSRI": S. Rako, 2000.

p.69 "Based on a Chinese parable": L. Kou, 1976.

p.71 "Gloria Steinem, in an interview": C. Dreifus, 1999.

p.72 "Interviewed by Barbara Walters": Burelle's transcript of ABC's *20/20,* 2001.

p.73 "A Swedish study": L. Bergkvist, 1989.

p.73 "along with publications by a group of researchers": R. K. Ross, 2000 (both listings).

p.73 "customarily prescribe some regimen of progestin": P. J. Sulak, 1997.

p.73 "They are investigating ways to shut down the menstrual cycle": M. Gladwell, 2000 (second listing).

p.74 "reports of women 'overdosing' with progesterone cream": E. F. Ilyia, 1998.

p.74 "even two to four times the manufacturer's recommended amount": A. Cooper, 1998.

p.74 "A recent study by researchers in the United Kingdom": K. Wyatt, 2001.

p.75 "abnormal levels of cycling hormones do not cause PMS": P. J. Schmidt, 1998.

p.75 "A small dose of Zoloft (sertraline)": D. M. Jermain, 1999.

p.76 "sometimes have a very tough time": P. J. Sulak, 1997.

p.76 "the Women's Health Initiative": Writing Group for the Women's Health Initiative Investigators, 2002.

p.77 "'PEPI'": Writing Group for the PEPI, 1995, 1996.

p.77 "'HERS'": S. Hulley, 1998.

p.77 "'The Time Has Come'": M. E. Mendelsohn, 2001.

p.83 "progesterone stimulates cell division in the breast": M. C. Pike, 1984.

p.83 "progesterone slows the clearance of estrogen": E. L. Klaiber, 1997; V. M. Jassoni, 1983.

p.84 "the beneficial effects of estrogen on our heart and blood vessels": J-F Arnal, 2001.

5. Medical Experiments and My Father's Hat

p.89 "I had no difficulty finding": E. M. Coutinho, 1966.

p.89 "In the Introduction to": E. M. Coutinho, 1999.

p.90 "I found in the archives": E. M. Coutinho, 1982.

p.96 "For any who want to look at the studies": W. G. Wiest, 1970; A. I. Csapo, 1971.

6. The Truth About "The Shot"

p.100 "the shot was not approved for marketing": C. E. Chilvers, 1996.

p.100 "to cause malignant mammary tumors": C. Paul, 1989.

p.100 "A 1995 analysis of the data": D. C. G. Skegg, 1995.

p.100 "'should be advised of the possibility'": C. E. Chilvers, 1996; D. C. G. Skegg, 1995.

p.100 "'the shot' appears neither to increase nor": The WHO Collaborative Study, 1991 (second listing), 1992.

p.101 "The physiology of bone growth": A. M. Parfitt, 1987; H. Haapasalo, 1996.

p.101 "the strongest our bones will ever be—by the time we are twenty": H. Haapasalo, 1996.

p.102 "A 1996 editorial": V. Matkovic, 1996.

p.102 "that girls attempt to delay the onset": E. M. Coutinho, 1999.

p.102 "with potentially serious consequences": B. A. Cromer, 1996; T. Cundy, 1991.

p.102 "A profoundly important study": B. A. Cromer, 1996.

p.103 **"Young women develop old women's bones":** W. B. Cutler, *No More Periods?* 2003 (Letter).

p.103 "The New Zealand studies and several others": T. Cundy, 1991,

1998; D. Scholes, 1999; L. C. Paiva, 1998; A. B. Berenson, 2001; A. M. Kaunitz, 1999; D. B. Petitti, 2000.

p.103 **"'Use of DMPA (Depo-Provera) should be considered a potential risk factor'":** T. Cundy, 1991.

p.104 "reported the case of a '33-year-old healthy, active woman'": G. J. Harkins, 1999.

p.105 "bone density loss 'appears reversible'": A. M. Kaunitz, 1999; D. B. Petitti, 2000.

p.105 "does damage to bone that cannot be remedied *even with discontinuation*": V. Matkovic, 1996; T. Cundy, 1998; D. Scholes, 1999.

p.105 *"is its undesirable effect on blood cholesterol":* World Health Organization, 1993.

p.106 "Most women spot and bleed": C. Paul, 1997.

p.107 "a particular set of neurons tends to accumulate": H. D. Rees, 1986.

p.107 "A Milwaukee study": S. C. Matson, 1997.

p.107 "'and 60 girls from a private clinic'": C. Templeman, 2000.

p.107 "One study that described': A. J. Davis, 1996.

p.107 "Adult women who use Depo-Provera gain weight, too": A. Nelson, 1996; C. Paul, 1997.

p.107 "'was an important reason for stopping'": C. Paul, 1997.

p.107 "also reported weight gain as a common reason": H. Sangi-Haghpeykar, 1996.

p.108 "'overall, 56% [of the users] reported less interest in sex'": Z. Harel, 1995.

p.108 "Here is one case study": A. M. Kaunitz, 1999.

p.110 "the average time to return to fertility is ten months": A. Nelson, 1996.

p.110 "Reports of the depressive effects": A. Nelson, 1996; D. Civic, 2000; E. L. Klaiber, 2001.

p.110 "One of the studies I read confirmed": D. Civic, 2000.

p.110 **"Headaches:** the most common side effect": A. Nelson, 1996.

p.110 **"Abdominal distress/pain":** R. S. Fisher, 1978; F. L. Datz, 1987.

p.110 "a decreased risk of benign fibroid tumors": P. Lumbiganon, 1996.

p.110 "A website that has accumulated": http://htmlgear.lycos.com/ guest/control.guest?u=shellyborsits&i=1&a=view

7. The More-or-Less Nonstop Birth Control Pill

p.115 "at least ten million American women": L. J. Piccinino, 1998.

p.116 "Women who regularly experience severe migraine headaches": K. Digre, 1987; S. D. Silberstein, 1991, 1992.

p.116 "Some women's migraine headaches are made worse": B. W. Somerville, 1972.

p.116 "Women with a seizure disorder": T. Bäckström, 1976, 1984; S. Duncan, 1993; A. G. Herzog, 1995, 1997; G. L. Holmes, 1988; P. Klein, 1998; R. H. Mattson, 1981; A. W. Zimmerman, 1986.

p.117 "the Pill can substantially (up to 50 percent) reduce": R. B. Ness, 2000; J. L. Stanford, 1991; The Cancer and Steroid Hormone Study, 1987; S. E. Hankinson, 1995; A. S. Whittemore, 1992.

p.117 "Between 1973 and 1982, as it became apparent": W. D. Mosher, 1990.

p.118 "condom use has increased": W. D. Mosher, 1990.

p.118 "'the most commonly reported method of contraception'": L. J. Piccinino, 1998.

p.119 "experimenting with a variety of hormone formulas": S. R. Killick, 1998; J. Rowan, 1999.

p.120 "which ties up our body's available testosterone": J. Nathorst-Boos, 1993; J. Bancroft, 1991; A. A. Murphy, 1990.

p.120 "Reduced levels of available testosterone": S. Rako, 1999; C. A. Graham, 1993; N. L. McCoy, 1996; P. Warner, 1988.

p.121 "with damaging consequences to a woman's immune and stress responses": M. Fern, 1978; K. L. Klove, 1984; C. Kirschbaum, 1995, 1996, 1999.

p.121 " 'Oral contraceptive users compared to nonusers' ": J. M. Scanlan, 1995.

p.121 "also demonstrated 'an increased incidence of self-reported illness' ": J. M. Scanlan, 1995.

p.121 " 'and are less well equipped to cope' ": A. T. Masi, 1995.

p.122 *"Many women still view menstruation"*: E. M. Coutinho, 1999.

p.122 "to have NO withdrawal bleed": M. D. G. Gillmer, 1978.

p.123 "with resulting suppression of sexual interest and response": C. A. Graham, 1993; P. Warner, 1988; S. Rako, 1999.

p.124 *"she benefits from a protective cyclic reduction in blood pressure"*: V. H. Moran, 2000.

p.124 *"Even small increases in blood pressure"*: R. L. Prentice, 1988.

p.125 "to be at increased risk of developing blood clots": J. I. Mann, 1975; H. W. Ory, 1977.

p.125 "a twenty-five-year followup of forty-six thousand women": V. Beral, 1999.

p.125 *"It is now established that in addition"*: B. V. Stadel, 1981.

p.126 "the risk of fatal pulmonary embolism": F. R. Rosendaal, 2002; W. O. Spitzer, 1996.

p.127 "a life-threatening condition known as pulmonary embolism": F. R. Rosendaal, 2002; W. O. Spitzer, 1996; N. Weiss, 1995; World Health Organization, 1995.

p.127 *"Because oral contraceptives are so widely used"*: F. R. Rosendaal, 2002.

p.129 "'an urgent public health issue that may affect millions'": I. Schiff, 1999.

p.129 "the conference of the Association of Reproductive Health Professionals": I. Schiff, 1999.

p.130 *"Although the incidence of fatal thromboembolism"*: H. Price, 1997.

p.131 "women who carry a gene called factor V Leiden": K. W. Bloemenkamp, 1995.

8. "The Pill" and the Virus That Causes Cancer

p.134 "a '25 year follow up of a cohort of 46,000 women'": V. Beral, 1999.

p.135 "an earlier U.K. study": M. P. Vessey, 1983.

p.135 "that implicated infection with the Humanpapilloma Virus": M. M. Madeleine, 2001; C. Ley, 1991.

p.136 "The connections are there, and they are worrisome": L. A. Brinton, 1986; World Health Organization, 1985; M. P. Vessey, 1983; M. M. Madeleine, 2001.

p.136 "The first paper was a 1986 publication": L. A. Brinton, 1986.

p.137 "By 1991, investigators were reporting": C. Ley, 1991.

p.137 "The most 'in your face' study": M. M. Madeleine, 2001.

9. The Sexiest Thing About a Woman

p.141 "women from all parts of the world have been writing":
http:www.mum.org/stopmen3.htm

References

Anderson, D. C., "Sex-hormone-binding Globulin," *Clinical Endocrinology* 3 (1974): 69–96.

Arbeit, J. M., P. M. Howley, and D. Hanahan, "Chronic Estrogen-induced Cervical and Vaginal Squamous Carcinogenesis in Human Papillomavirus Type 16 Transgenic Mice," *Proceedings of the National Academy of Science* 93 (1996): 2930–2935.

Archer, D. F., R. Maheux, A. DelConte, F. B. O'Brien, and the North American Levonorgestrel Study Group (NALSG), "A New Low-Dose Monophasic Combination Oral Contraceptive (Alesse) with Levonorgestrel 100 μg and Ethinyl Estradiol 20 μg," *Contraception* 55 (1997): 139–144.

Arnal, J-F, and F. Bayard, "Vasculoprotective Effects of Oestrogens," *Clinical and Experimental Pharmacology and Physiology* 28 (2001): 1032–1034.

Bachmann, G. A., "Androgen Cotherapy in Menopause: Evolving Benefits and Challenges," *American Journal of Obstetrics and Gynecology* 180 (1999): S308–S311.

Bachrach, C. A., "Contraceptive Practice Among American Women, 1973–1982," *Family Planning Perspectives,* 16, no. 6 (1984): 253–259.

Bäckström, T., "Epileptic Seizures in Women Related to Plasma Estrogen and Progesterone During the Menstrual Cycle," *Acta Neurologica Scandinavia* 54 (1976): 321–347.

Bäckström, T., B. Zetterlund, S. Blom, and M. Romano, "Effects of Intravenous Progesterone Infusions on the Epileptic Discharge Frequency in Women with Partial Epilepsy," *Acta Neurologica Scandinavia* 69 (1984): 240–248.

Bancroft, J., B. B. Sherwin, G. M. Alexander, D. W. Davidson, and A. Walker, "Oral Contraceptives, Androgens, and the Sexuality of Young Women: II. The Role of Androgens," *Archives of Sexual Behavior* 20, no. 2 (1991): 121–135.

Barrett-Connor, E., "Efficacy and Safety of Estrogen/Androgen Therapy. Menopausal Symptoms, Bone, and Cardiovascular Parameters," *Journal of Reproductive Medicine* 43, no. 8/Supplement (1998): 746–752.

Beral, V., C. Hermon, C. Kay, P. Hannaford, S. Darby, and G. Reeves, "Mortality Associated with Oral Contraceptive Use: 25 Year Follow Up of Cohort of 46,000 Women from Royal College of General Practitioners' Oral Contraception Study," *British Medical Journal* 318 (January 9, 1999): 96–100.

Berenson, A. B., C. M. Radecki, J. J. Grady, V. I. Rickert, and A. Thomas, "A Prospective, Controlled Study of the Effects of Hormonal Contraception on Bone Mineral Density," *Obstetrics and Gynecology* 98, no. 4 (2001): 576–582.

Bergkvist, L., H. O. Adami, I. Persson, R. Hoover, and C. Schairer, "The Risk of Breast Cancer After Estrogen and Estrogen-Progestin Replacement," *The New England Journal of Medicine* 321 (1989): 293–297.

Bloemenkamp, K. W., F. R. Rosendall, F. M. Helmerhorst, H. R. Buller, and J. P. Vandenbroucke, "Enhancement by Factor V Leiden Mutation of Risk of Deep-vein Thrombosis Associated with Oral Contraceptives Containing a Third-generation Progestagen," *The Lancet* 346 (December 16, 1995): 1593–1596.

Brinton, L. A., G. R. Huggins, H. F. Lehman, K. Mallin, D. A. Savitz, E. Trapido, J. Rosenthal, and R. Hoover, "Long-term Use of Oral Contraceptives and Risk of Invasive Cervical Cancer," *International Journal of Cancer* 38 (1986): 339–344.

Brown, B. G., X. Q. Zhao, A. Chait, L. D. Fisher, M. C. Cheung, J. S. Morse, A. A. Dowdy, E. K. Marino, E. L. Bolson, P. Alaupovic, J. Frohlich, L. Serafini, E. Huss-Frechette, S. Wang, D. DeAngelis, A. Dodek, and J. J. Albers, "Simvastatin and Niacin, Antioxidant Vitamins, or the Combination for the Prevention of Coronary Disease," *New England Journal of Medicine* 345, no. 22 (2001): 1583–1592.

Burelle's Information Services transcription of ABC's *20/20, Barbara Walters' Interview with Gloria Steinem* (Item # 10330): Friday, March 30, 2001.

The Cancer and Steroid Hormone Study of the Centers for Disease Control and the National Institute of Child Health and Human Development, "The Reduction in Risk of Ovarian Cancer Associated with Oral-Contraceptive Use," *New England Journal of Medicine* 316 (March 12, 1987): 650–655.

Carr, B. R., C. R. Parker, J. D. Madden, P. C. MacDonald, and J. C. Porter, "Plasma Levels of Adrenocorticotropin and Cortisol in Women Receiving Oral Contraceptive Steroid Treatment," *Journal of Clinical Endocrinology and Metabolism* 49, no. 3 (1979): 346–349.

Chilvers, C. E., "Depot Medroxyprogesterone Acetate and Breast Cancer," *Drug Safety* 15, no. 3 (1996): 212–218.

Civic, D., D. Scholes, L. Ichikawa, A. Z. LaCroix, C. K. Yoshida, S. M. Ott, and W. E. Barlow, "Depressive Symptoms in Users and Non-Users of Depot Medroxyprogesterone Acetate," *Contraception* 61 (2000): 385–390.

Collaborative Group on Hormonal Factors in Breast Cancer, "Breast Cancer and Hormonal Contraceptives: Collaborative Reanalysis of Individual Data on 53,297 Women with Breast Cancer and 100,239 Women without Breast Cancer from 54 Epidemiological Studies," *The Lancet* 347 (June 22, 1996): 1713–1727.

Cook, J. D., and E. R. Monsen, "Food Iron Absorption. I. Use of a Semisynthetic Diet to Study Absorption of Nonheme Iron," *American Journal of Clinical Nutrition* 28 (1975): 1289–1295.

Cooper, A., C. Spencer, M. I. Whitehead, D. Ross, C. J. R. Barnard, and W. P. Collins, "Systemic Absorption of Progesterone from Progest Cream in Postmenopausal Women," *The Lancet* 351 (April 25, 1998): 1255–1256.

Coutinho, E. M., "Kaposi's Sarcoma and the Use of Oestrogen by Male Homosexuals," *The Lancet* (June 12, 1982): 1362.

Coutinho, E. M., J. C. De Souza, and A. I. Csapo, "Reversible Sterility Induced by Medroxyprogesterone Injections," *Fertility and Sterility* 17, no. 2 (1966): 261–266.

Coutinho, E. M., A. R. da Silva, C. E. Mattos, N. C. Nielsen, M. Osler, and J. Wiese, "Contraception with Long Acting Subdermal Implants: I. An Effective and Acceptable Modality in International Clinical Trials," *Contraception* 18, no. 4 (1978): 315–333.

Coutinho, E. M., J. C. De Souza, C. Athayde, I. C. Barbosa, F. Alvarez, V. Brache, G. Zhi-Ping, E. E. Emuveyan, A. O. Adekunle, L. Devoto, M. M. Shaaban, H. T. Salem, B. Affandi, O. Mateo de Acosta, J. Mati, and O. A. Ladipo, "Multicenter Clinical Trial on the Efficacy and Acceptability of a Single Contraceptive Implant of Monegestrol Acetate, Uniplant," *Contraception* 53 (1996): 121–125.

Coutinho, E. M., I. Mascarenhas, O. M. Acosta, J. G. Flores, Z-P. Gu, O. A. Ladipo, A. O. Adekunle, E. O. Otolorin, M. M. Shaaban, M. A. Oyoon, A. Kamal, A. Plah, N. C. Sikazwe, and S. J. Segal, "Comparative Study on the Efficacy, Acceptability, and Side Effects of a Contraceptive Pill Administered by the Oral and the Vaginal Route: An International Multicenter Clinical Trial," *Clinical Pharmacology & Therapeutics* 54, no. 5 (1993): 540–545.

Coutinho, E. M., and S. J. Segal, *Is Menstruation Obsolete?* New York: Oxford University Press, 1999.

Coutinho, E. M., P. Spinola, I. Barbosa, M. Gatto, G. Tomaz, K. Morais, M. E. Yazlle, R. N. de Souza, J. S. P. Neto, W. de Barros Leal, C. Leal, S. B. Hippolito, and A. D. Abranches, "Multicenter, Double-blind, Comparative Clinical Study on the Efficacy and Acceptability of a Monthly Injectable Contraceptive Combination of 150 mg Dihydroxyprogesterone Acetophenide and 10 mg Estradiol Enanthate Compared to a Monthly Injectable Contraceptive Combination of 90 mg Dihydroxyprogesterone Acetophenide and 6 mg Estradiol Enanthate," *Contraception* 55 (1997): 175–181.

Cromer, B. A., "Recent Clinical issues Related to the Use of Depot Medroxyprogesterone Acetate (Depo-Provera)," *Current Opinion in Obstetrics and Gynecology* 11, no. 5 (1999): 467–471.

Cromer, B. A., J. M. Blair, J. D. Mahan, L. Zibners, and Z. Naumovski, "A Prospective Comparison of Bone Density in Adolescent Girls Receiving Depot Medroxyprogesterone Acetate (Depo-Provera), Levonorgestrel (Norplant), or Oral Contraceptives," *Journal of Pediatrics* 129, no. 5 (1996): 671–676.

Csapo, A. I., J. Sauvage, and W. G. Wiest, "The Efficacy and Acceptability of Intravenously Administered Prostaglandin F $_{2\alpha}$ as an Abortifacient," *American Journal of Obstetrics and Gynecology* 111 (1971): 1059–1063.

Cundy, T., J. Cornish, H. Roberts, H. Elder, and I. R. Reid, "Spinal Bone Density in Women Using Depot Medroxyprogesterone Contraception," *Obstetrics and Gynecology* 92, no. 4/part 1 (1998): 569–573.

Cundy, T., M. Evans, H. Roberts, D. Wattie, R. Ames, and I. R. Reid, "Bone Density in Women Receiving Depot Medroxyprogesterone Acetate for Contraception," *British Medical Journal* 303 (July 6, 1991): 13–16.

Cutler, W. B., *Love Cycles: The Science of Intimacy.* Haverford, Pennsylvania: Athena Institute Press, 1991.

Cutler, W. B., "Letter," *No More Periods? The Risks of Menstrual Suppression and Other Cutting-Edge Issues About Hormones and Women's Health,* Rako, S. New York: Harmony Books, 2003.

Cutler, W. B., C. R. Garcia, G. R. Huggins, and G. Preti, "Sexual Behavior and Steroid Levels Among Gynecologically Mature Premenopausal Women," *Fertility and Sterility* 45, no. 4 (1986): 496–502.

Cutler, W. B., C. R. Garcia, and A. M. Krieger, "Sexual Behavior Frequency and Menstrual Cycle Length in Mature Premenopausal Women," *Psychoneuroendocrinology* 4, no. 4 (1979): 297–309.

Cutler, W. B., C. R. Garcia, and A. M. Krieger, "Luteal Phase Defects: A Possible Relationship Between Short Hyperthermic Phase and Sporadic Sexual Behavior in Women," *Hormones & Behavior* 13, no. 3 (1979): 214–218.

Cutler, W. B., G. Preti, G. Huggins, B. Erickson, and C. R. Garcia, "Sexual Behavior Frequency and Biphasic Ovulatory Type Menstrual Cycles," *Physiology & Behavior* 34, no. 5 (1985): 805–810.

Cutler, W. B., G. Preti, A. Krieger, G. R. Huggins, C. R. Garcia, and H. J. Lawley, "Human Axillary Secretions Influence Women's Menstrual Cycles: The Role of Donor Extract from Men," *Hormonal Behavior* 20, no. 4 (1986): 463–473.

Datz, F. L., P. E. Christian, and J. Moore, "Gender-Related Differences in Gastric Emptying," *Journal of Nuclear Medicine* 28 (1987): 1204–1207.

Davidoff, F., C. D. DeAngelis, J. M. Drazen, J. Hoey, L. Hojgaard, R. Horton, S. Kotzin, M. G. Nicholls, M. Nylenna, J. P. M. Overbeke, H. C. Sox, M. B. Van Der Weyden, and M. S. Wilkes, "Sponsorship, Authorship, and Accountability," *Journal of the American Medical Association* 286, no. 10 (September 12, 2001).

Davidoff, F., C. D. DeAngelis, J. M. Drazen, J. Hoey, L. Hojgaard, R. Horton, S. Kotzin, M. G. Nicholls, M. Nylenna, J. P. M. Overbeke, H. C. Sox, M. B. Van Der Weyden, and M. S. Wilkes, "Sponsorship, Authorship, and Accountability," *Obstetrics and Gynecology* 98, no. 6 (2001): 1143–1146.

Davidoff, F., C. D. DeAngelis, J. M. Drazen, J. Hoey, L. Hojgaard, R. Horton, S. Kotzin, M. G. Nicholls, M. Nylenna, J. P. M. Overbeke, H. C. Sox, M. B. Van Der Weyden, and M. S. Wilkes, "Sponsorship, Authorship, and Accountability," *The Lancet* 358, no. 9285 (2001): 854–856.

Davidoff, F., C. D. DeAngelis, J. M. Drazen, J. Hoey, L. Hojgaard, R. Horton, S. Kotzin, M. G. Nicholls, M. Nylenna, J. P. M. Overbeke, H. C. Sox, M. B. Van Der Weyden, and M. S. Wilkes, "Sponsorship, Authorship, and Accountability," *Annals of Internal Medicine* 135, no. 6 (2001): 463–466.

Davis, A. J., "Use of Depot Medroxyprogesterone Acetate Contraception in Adolescents," *Journal of Reproductive Medicine* 41/ Supplement (1996): 407–413.

Davis, S., "Androgen Replacement in Women: A Commentary," *Journal of Clinical Endocrinology and Metabolism* 84, no. 6 (1999): 1886–1891.

Davis, S. R., P. McCloud, B. J. G. Strauss, and H. Burger, "Testosterone Enhances Estradiol's Effects on Postmenopausal Bone Density and Sexuality," *Maturitas* 21 (1995): 227–236.

de Valk, B., and J. J. M. Marx, "Iron, Atherosclerosis, and Ischemic Heart Disease," *Archives of Internal Medicine* 159 (July 26, 1999): 1542–1548.

Digre, K., and H. Damasio, "Menstrual Migraine: Differential Diagnosis, Evaluation, and Treatment," *Clinical Obstetrics and Gynecology* 30, no. 2 (1987): 417–430.

Dreifus, C., *Modern Maturity,* June 1999. Interview with Gloria Steinem.

Duncan, S., C. L. Read, and M. J. Brodie, "How Common Is Catamenial Epilepsy?" *Epilepsia* 34, no. 5 (1993): 827–831.

Eklund, A. C., M. M. Belchak, K. Lapidos, R. Raha-Chowdhury, and C. Ober, "Polymorphisms in the HLA-linked Olfactory Receptor Genes in the Hutterites," *Human Immunology* 61, no. 7 (2000): 711–717.

Farmer, R. D. T., and R. A. Lawrenson, "Third Generation Oral Contraceptives and Venous Thrombosis," *The Lancet* 349 (1995): 732–773.

Fern, M., D. P. Rose, and E. B. Fern, "Effect of Oral Contraceptives on Plasma Androgenic Steroids and Their Precursors," *Obstetrics and Gynecology* 51, no. 5 (1978): 541–544.

Feskanich, D., V. Singh, W. C. Willett, and G. A. Colditz, "Vitamin A Intake and Hip Fractures Among Postmenopausal Women," *Journal of the American Medical Association* 287 (January 2, 2002): 47–54.

Fisch, I. R., and J. Frank, "Oral Contraceptives and Blood Pressure," *Journal of the American Medical Association* 237, no. 23 (1977): 2499–2503.

Fisher, R. S., G. S. Roberts, C. J. Grabowski, and S. Cohen, "Inhibition of Lower Esophageal Sphincter Circular Muscle by Female Sex Hormones," *American Journal of Physiology* 234, no. 3 (1978): E243–E247.

Fletcher, S. W., and G. A. Colditz, "Failure of Estrogen Plus Progestin Therapy for Prevention," *Journal of the American Medical Association* 288 (July 17, 2002): 366–368.

Francis-Cheung, T., *A Break in Your Cycle.* Minneapolis, Minnesota: Chronimed Publishers, 1998.

Gillmer, M. D., E. J. Fox, and H. S. Jacobs, "Failure of Withdrawal Bleeding During Combined Oral Contraceptive Therapy: 'Amenorrhoea on the Pill,' " *Contraception* 18, no. 5 (1978): 507–515.

Gladwell, M., "John Rock's Error," *The New Yorker,* March 13, 2000: 52–63.

Gladwell, M., *The Tipping Point.* Boston, New York, London: Little, Brown and Company, 2000.

Graham, C. A., and B. B. Sherwin, "The Relationship Between Mood and Sexuality in Women Using an Oral Contraceptive as a Treatment for Premenstrual Symptoms," *Psychoendocrinology* 18, no. 4 (1993): 273–281.

Grady, D., S. M. Rubin, D. B. Betitti, C. S. Fox, D. Black, B. Ettinger, V. L. Ernster, and S. R. Cummings, "Hormone Therapy to Prevent Disease and Prolong Life in Postmenopausal Women," *Annals of Internal Medicine* 117, no. 12 (1992): 1016–1037.

Grant, E. C. G., "Dangers of Suppressing Menstruation," *The Lancet* 356 (August 5, 2000): 513–514.

Grant, E. C. G., and J. Pryse-Davies, "Effect of Oral Contraceptives on Depressive Mood Changes and on Endometrial Monoamine Oxidase and Phosphatases," *British Medical Journal* 3 (1968): 777.

Haapasalo, H., P. Kannus, H. Sievänen, M. Pasanen, K. Uusi-Rasi, A. Heinonen, P. Oja, and I. Vuori, "Development of Mass, Density, and Estimated Mechanical Characteristics of Bones in Caucasian Females," *Journal of Bone and Mineral Research* 11, no. 11 (1996): 1751–1760.

Halbreich, U., N. Rojansky, and S. Palter, "Elimination of Ovulation and Menstrual Cyclicity (with Danazol) Improves Dysphoric Premenstrual Syndromes," *Fertility and Sterility* 56 (1991): 1066.

Hankinson, S. E., G. A. Colditz, D. J. Hunter, W. C. Willett, M. J. Stampfer, B. Rosner, C. H. Hennekens, and F. E. Speizer, "A Prospective Study of Reproductive Factors and Risk of Epithelial Ovarian Cancer," *Cancer* 76 (1995): 284–290.

Harel, Z., F. M. Biro, and L. M. Kollar, "Depo-Provera in Adolescents: Effects of Early Second Injection or Prior Oral Contraception," *Journal of Adolescent Health* 16, no. 5 (1995): 379–384.

Harkins, G. J., G. D. Davis, J. Dettori, M. L. Hibbert, and R. A. Hoyt, "Decline in Bone Mineral Density with Stress Fractures in a Woman on Depot Medroxyprogesterone Acetate," *Journal of Reproductive Medicine* 44 (1999): 309–312.

Herzberg, B. N., A. L. Johnson, and S. Brown, "Depressive Symptoms and Oral Contraceptives," *British Medical Journal* 4 (1970): 142.

Herzog, A. G., "Progesterone Therapy in Women with Complex Partial and Secondary Generalized Seizures," *Neurology* 45 (1995): 1660–1662.

Herzog, A. G., P. Klein, and B. J. Ransil, "Three Patterns of Catamenial Epilepsy," *Epilepsia* 38, no. 10 (1997): 1082–1088.

Hildesheim, A., W. C. Reeves, L. A. Brinton, C. Lavery, M. Brenes, M. E. De La Guardia, J. Godoy, and W. E. Rawls, "Association of Oral Contraceptive Use and Human Papillomaviruses in Invasive Cervical Cancers," *International Journal of Cancer* 45 (1990): 860–864.

Hill, J. S., M. R. Hayden, J. Frohlich, and P. H. Pritchard, "Genetic and Environmental Factors Affecting the Incidence of Coronary Artery Disease in Heterozygous Familial Hypercholesterolemia," *Arteriosclerosis and Thrombosis* 11 (1991): 290–297.

Holmes, G. L., "Effects of Menstruation and Pregnancy on Epilepsy," *Seminars in Neurology* 8, no. 3 (1988): 234–239.

Hu, F. B., M. J. Stampfer, J. E. Manson, F. Grodstein, G. A. Colditz, F. E. Speizer, and W. C. Willett, "Trends in the Incidence of Coronary Heart Disease and Changes in Diet and Lifestyle in Women," *New England Journal of Medicine* 343 (August 24, 2000): 530–537.

Hulley, S., D. Grady, T. Bush, C. Furberg, D. Herrington, B. Riggs, and E. Vittinghoff, for the Heart and Estrogen-progestin Replacement Study (HERS) Research Group, "Randomized Trial of Estrogen Plus Progestin for Secondary Prevention of Coronary Heart Disease in Postmenopausal Women," *Journal of the American Medical Association* 280 (August 19, 1998): 605–613.

Ilyia, E. F., D. McLure, and M. Y. Farhat, "Topical Progesterone Cream Application and Overdosing," *Journal of Alternative and Complementary Medicine* 4, no. 1 (1998): 5–6.

Jacob, S., M. K. McClintock, B. Zelano, and C. Ober, "Paternally Inherited HLA Alleles Are Associated with Women's Choice of Male Odor," *Nature Genetics* 30, no. 2 (2002): 175–179.

Jasonni, V. M., C. Bulletti, F. Franceschetti, P. Ciotti, M. Bonavia, A. P. Ferraretti, and C. Flamigni, "Preliminary Report on Progesterone Effect on Peripheral Estrone Sulfate Metabolism," *Acta European Fertility* 14, no. 2 (1983): 137–140.

Jensen, J., B. J. Riis, B. Strom, L. Nilas, and C. Christiansen, "Long-Term Effects of Percutaneous Estrogens and Oral Progesterone on Serum Liproproteins in Postmenopausal Women," *American Journal of Obstetrics and Gynecology* 156, no. 1 (1987): 66–71.

Jermain, D. M., C. K. Preece, R. L. Sykes, T. J. Kuehl, and P. J. Sulak, "Luteal Phase Sertraline Treatment for Premenstrual Dysphoric Disorder. Results of a Double-blind, Placebo-Controlled, Crossover Study," *Archives of Family Medicine* 8 (1999): 328–332.

Karlson, P., and M. Luscher, "Pheromones: A new term for biologically active substances," *Nature* 4653 (1959): 55–56.

Kaunitz, A. M., "Long-acting Injectable Contraception with Depot Medroxyprogesterone Acetate," *American Journal of Obstetrics and Gynecology* 170, no. 5/part 2 (1994): 1543–1549.

Kaunitz, A. M., "Injectable Depot Medroxyprogesterone Acetate Contraception: An Update for U.S. Clinicians," *International Journal of Fertility and Women's Medicine* 43, no. 2 (1998): 73–83.

Kaunitz, A. M., "Long-acting Hormonal Contraception: Assessing Impact on Bone Density, Weight, and Mood," *International Journal of Fertility* 44, no. 2 (1999): 110–117.

Kiechl, S., J. Willeit, G. Egger, W. Poewe, and F. Oberhollenzer, "Body Iron Stores and the Risk of Carotid Atherosclerosis," *Circulation* 96 (1997): 3300–3307.

Killick, S. R., C. Fitzgerald, and A. Davis, "Ovarian Activity in Women Taking an Oral Contraceptive Containing 20 µg Ethinyl Estradiol and 150 µg Desogestrel: Effects of Low Estrogen Doses During the Hormone-free Interval," *American Journal of Obstetrics and Gynecology* 179, no. 1 (1998): S18–24.

Kirschbaum, C., B. M. Kudielka, J. Gaab, N. C. Schommer, and D. H. Hellhammer, "Impact of Gender, Menstrual Cycle Phase, and Oral Contraceptives on the Activity of the Hypothalamus–pituitary–adrenal axis," *American Psychosomatic Society* 61 (1999): 154–162.

Kirschbaum, C., K-M. Pirke, and D. H. Hellhammer, "Preliminary Evidence for Reduced Cortisol Responsivity to Psychological Stress in Women Using Oral Contraceptive Medication," *Psychoneuroendocrinology* 20, no. 5 (1995): 509–514.

Kirschbaum, C., P. Platte, K-M. Pirke, and D. H. Hellhammer, "Adrenocortical Activation Following Stressful Exercise: Further Evidence for Attenuated Free Cortisol Responses in Women Using Oral Contraceptives," *Stress Medicine* 12 (1996): 137–143.

Klaiber, E. L., *Hormones and the Mind*. New York: HarperCollins, 2001.

Klaiber, E. L., D. M. Broverman, W. Vogel, L. G. Peterson, and M. B. Snyder, "Relationships of Serum Estradiol Levels, Menopausal Duration, and Mood During Hormonal Replacement Therapy," *Psychoneuroendocrinology* 22, no. 7 (1997): 549–558.

Klein, P., and A. G. Herzog, "Hormonal Effects on Epilepsy in Women," *Epilepsia* 39/Supplement 8 (1998): S9–S16.

Kleiner, S. M., "Antioxidant Answers," *Physician and Sports Medicine* 24, no. 8 (August 1996).

Klove, K. L., S. Roy, and R. A. Lobo, "The Effect of Different Contraceptive Treatments on the Serum Concentration of Dehydroepiandrosterone Sulfate," *Contraception* 29, no. 4 (1984): 319–324.

Kou, L., and Y-H. Kou, *Chinese Folk Tales*, Millbrae, California: Celestial Arts, 1976, pp. 83–85.

Kurunmäki, H., J. Toivonen, P. Lähteenmäki, and T. Luukkainen, "Intracervical Release of Levonorgestrel for Contraception," *Contraception* 23 (1981): 473.

Kushi, L. H., A. R. Folsom, R. J. Prineas, P. J. Mink, Y. Wu, and R. M. Bostick, "Dietary Antioxidant Vitamins and Death from Coronary Heart Disease in Postmenopausal Women," *New England Journal of Medicine* 334, no. 18 (1996): 1156–1162.

Lacey, J. V., P. J. Mink, J. H. Lubin, M. E. Sherman, R. Troisi, P. Hartge, A. Schatzkin, and C. Schairer, "Menopausal Hormone Replacement Therapy and Risk of Ovarian Cancer," *Journal of the American Medical Association* 288 (July 17, 2002): 334–341.

Ley, C., H. M. Bauer, A. Reingold, M. H. Schiffman, J. C. Chambers, C. J. Tashiro, and M. M. Manos, "Determinants of Genital Human Papillomavirus Infection in Young Women," *Journal of the National Cancer Institute* 83, no. 14 (1991): 997–1003.

Lipman, M. M., F. H. Katz, and J. W. Jailer, "An Alternate Pathway for Cortisol Metabolism: 6β-hydroxy-cortisol Production by Human Tissue Slices," *Journal of Endocrinology and Metabolism* 22 (1962): 268–272.

Lumbiganon, P., S. Rugpao, S. Phandu-fung, M. Laopaiboon, N. Vudhikamraksa, and Y. Werawatakul, "Protective Effect of Depot-Medroxyprogesterone Acetate on Surgically Treated Uterine Leiomyomas: A Multicentre Case-control Study," *British Journal of Obstetrics and Gynaecology* 103 (1996): 909–914.

Madeleine, M. M., J. R. Daling, S. M. Schwartz, K. Shera, B. McKnight, J. J. Carter, G. C. Wipf, C. W. Critchlow, J. K. McDougall, P. Porter, and D. A. Galloway, "Human Papillomavirus and Long-term Oral Contraceptive Use Increase the Risk of Adenocarcinoma *in Situ* of the Cervix," *Cancer Epidemiology, Biomarkers and Prevention* 10 (March 2001): 171–177.

Mann, J. I., M. P. Vessey, M. Thorogood, and R. Doll, "Myocardial Infarction in Young Women with Special Reference to Oral Contraceptive Practice," *British Medical Journal* 2 (1975): 241–245.

Masi, A. T., S. L. Feigenbaum, and R. T. Chatterton, "Hormonal and Pregnancy Relationships to Rheumatoid Arthritis: Convergent Effects with Immunologic and Microvascular Systems," *Seminars in Arthritis and Rheumatism* 25, no. 1 (1995): 1–27.

Matkovic, V., "Editorial: Skeletal Development and Bone Turnover Revisited," *Journal of Clinical Endocrinology and Metabolism* 81, no. 6 (1996): 2013–2016.

Matson, S. C., K. A. Henderson, and G. J. McGrath, "Physical Findings and Symptoms of Depot Medroxyprogesterone Acetate Use in Adolescent Females," *Journal of Pediatric and Adolescent Gynecology* 10 (1997): 18–23.

Mattson, R. H., J. A. Kamer, J. A. Cramer, and B. V. Caldwell, "Seizure Frequency and the Menstrual Cycle: A Clinical Study," *Epilepsia* 22 (1981): 242.

Mays, E. T., W. M. Christopherson, M. M. Mahr, and H. C. Williams, "Hepatic Changes in Young Women Ingesting Contraceptive Steroids: Hepatic Hemorrhage and Primary Hepatic Tumors," *Journal of the American Medical Association* 235, no. 7 (February 16, 1976): 730–732.

McClintock, M. K., "Menstrual Synchrony and Suppression," *Nature* 229 (1971): 244–245.

McCoy, N., W. Cutler, and J. M. Davidson, "Relationships Among Sexual Behavior, Hot Flashes, and Hormone Levels in Perimenopausal Women," *Archives of Sexual Behavior* 14, no. 5 (1985): 385–394.

McCoy, N. L., and M. A. Matyas, "Oral Contraceptives and Sexuality in University Women," *Archives of Sexual Behavior* 25, no. 1 (1996): 73–90.

Mendelsohn, M. E., and R. H. Karas, "The Time Has Come to Stop Letting the HERS Talc Wag the Dogma," *Circulation* 104 (November 6, 2001): 2256–2259.

Metzger, D. A., R. Chosak, J. Leventhal, and R. I. Young, "Practical Clinical Considerations in the Use of Estrogen/Androgen Therapy," *Journal of Reproductive Medicine* 43, no. 8/Supplement (1998): 753–762.

Meyers, D. G., D. Strickland, P. A. Maloley, J. J. Seburg, J. E. Wilson, and B. F. McManus, "Possible Association of a Reduction in Cardiovascular Events with Blood Donation," *Heart* 78 (1997): 188–193.

Miller, L., "Continuous Administration of 100 μg Levonorgestrel and 20 μg Ethinyl Estradiol for Elimination of Menses: A Randomized Trial," *Obstetrics and Gynecology* 97/Supplement (2001): 16S.

Miller, L., D. L. Patton, A. Meier, S. S. Thwin, T. M. Hooton, and D. A. Eschenbach, "Depomedroxyprogesterone-induced Hypoestrogenism and Changes in Vaginal Flora and Epithelium," *Obstetrics and Gynecology* 96, no. 3 (2000): 431–439.

Mishell, D. R., "Pharmacokinetics of Depot Medroxyprogesterone Acetate Contraception," *Journal of Reproductive Medicine* 41, no. 5/Supplement (1996): 381–390.

Mishell, D. R., K. M. Kharma, I. H. Thorneycroft, and R. M. Nakamura, "Estrogenic Activity in Women Receiving an Injectable Progestogen for Contraception," *American Journal of Obstetrics and Gynecology* 113 (1972): 372.

Moore, T. J., *Prescription for Disaster,* New York: Dell, 1998.

Moorjani, S., A. Dupont, F. Labrie, B. De Lignieres, L. Cusan, P. Dupont, J. Mailloux, and P. J. Lupien, "Changes in Plasma Lipoprotein and Apolipoprotein Composition in Relation to Oral Versus Percutaneous Administration of Estrogen Alone or in Association with Utrogestan in Menopausal Women," *Journal of Clinical Endocrinology and Metabolism* 73, no. 2 (1991): 373–379.

Moran, V. H., H. L. Leathard, and J. Coley, "Cardiovascular Functioning During the Menstrual Cycle," *Clinical Physiology* 20, no. 6 (2000): 496–504.

Morrison, H. I., R. M. Semenciw, Y. Mao, and D. T. Wigle, "Serum Iron and Risk of Fatal Acute Myocardial Infarction," *Epidemiology* 5 (1994): 243–246.

Mosher, W. D., "Contraceptive Practice in the United States, 1982–1988," *Family Planning Perspectives* 22, no. 5 (September/October 1990): 198–205.

Motluk, A., "Scent of a Man," *New Scientist* 169, no. 2277 (October 2, 2001): 36.

Muldoon, M. F., S. B., Manuck, and K. A. Matthews, "Lowering Cholesterol Concentrations and Mortality: A Quantitative Review of Primary Prevention Trials," *British Medical Journal* 301 (August 11, 1990): 309–314.

Murphy, A. A., C. S. Cropp, B. S. Smith, R. T. Burkman, and H. A. Zacur, "Effect of Low-Dose Oral Contraceptive on Gonadotropins, Androgens, and Sex Hormone Binding Globulin in Nonhirsute Women," *Fertility and Sterility* 53, no. 1 (1990): 35–39.

Nathorst-Böös, J., B. von Schoultz, and K. Carlström, "Elective Ovarian Removal and Estrogen Replacement Therapy—Effects on Sexual Life, Psychological Well-Being and Androgen Status," *Journal of Psychosomatic and Obstetric Gynaecology* 14 (1993): 283–293.

Nelson, A., "Counseling Issues and Management of Side Effects for Women Using Depot Medroxyprogesterone Acetate Contraception," *Journal of Reproductive Medicine* 41/Supplement 5 (1996): 391–400.

Ness, R. B., J. A. Grisso, J. Klapper, J. J. Schlesselman, S. Silberzweig, R. Vergona, M. Morgan, and J. E. Wheeler, "Risk of Ovarian Cancer in Relation to Estrogen and Progestin Dose and Use Characteristics of Oral Contraceptives," *American Journal of Epidemiology* 152, no. 3 (2000): 233–241.

Noller, K. L., "Estrogen Replacement Therapy and Risk of Ovarian Cancer," *Journal of the American Medical Association* 288 (July 17, 2002): 368–369.

Ober, C., "The Maternal-Fetal Relationship in Human Pregnancy: An Immunogenetic Perspective," *Experiments in Clinical Immunogenetics* 9, no. 1 (1992): 1–14.

Ober, C., S. Elias, D. D. Kostyu, and W. W. Hauck, "Decreased Fecundability in Hutterite Couples Sharing HLA-DR," *American Journal of Human Genetics* 50, no. 1 (1992): 6–14.

Ober, C. L., A. O. Martin, J. L. Simpson, W. W. Hauch, D. B. Amos, D. D. Kostyu, M. Fotino, and F. H. Allen, Jr., "Shared HLA Antigens and Reproductive Performance Among Hutterites," *American Journal of Human Genetics* 35, no. 5 (1983): 994–1004.

Ober, C., J. L. Simpson, M. Ward, R. M. Radvany, R. Andersen, S. Elias, and R. Sabbagha, "Prenatal Effects of Maternal-Fetal HLA Compatibility," *American Journal of Reproductive Immunology and Microbiology* 15, no. 4 (1987): 141–149.

Ober, C., L. R. Weitkamp, N. Cox, H. Dytch, D. Kostyu, and S. Elias, "HLA and Mate Choice in Humans," *American Journal of Human Genetics* 61, no. 3 (1997): 497–504.

Omenn, G. S., G. Goodman, and M. Thornquist, "The Beta-Carotene and Retinal Efficacy Trial (CARET) for Chemoprevention of Lung Cancer in High Risk Populations: Smokers and Asbestos-Exposed Workers," *Cancer Research* 54, no. 7/Supplement (1994): 2038–2042.

Ornstein, D., and L. R. Zachariski, "Coronary Artery Disease in Men and Women," *New England Journal of Medicine* 31, no. 25 (December 16, 1999): 1933.

Ory, H. W., "Association Between Oral Contraceptives and Myocardial Infarction," *Journal of the American Medical Association* 237, no. 24 (1977): 2619–2622.

Paiva, L. C., A. M. Pinto-Neto, and A. Faundes, "Bone Density Among Long-term Users of Medroxyprogesterone Acetate as a Contraceptive," *Contraception* 58 (1998): 351–355.

Parfitt, A. M., "Bone Remodeling and Bone Loss: Understanding the Pathophysiology of Osteoporosis," *Clinical Obstetrics and Gynecology* 30, no. 4 (1987): 789–811.

Paul, C., D. C. G. Skegg, and G. F. S. Spears, "Depot Medroxy-progesterone (Depo-Provera) and Risk of Breast Cancer," *British Medical Journal* 299 (September 23, 1989): 759–762.

Paul, C., D. C. G. Skegg, and S. Williams, "Depot Medroxy-progesterone Acetate. Patterns of Use and Reasons for Discontinuation," *Contraception* 56 (1997): 209–214.

Penckofer, S., and D. Schwertz, "Improved Iron Status Parameters May Be a Benefit of Hormone Replacement Therapy," *Journal of Women's Health & Gender-Based Medicine* 9, no. 2 (2000): 141–151.

Petitti, D. B., G. Piaggio, S. Mehta, M. C. Cravioto, and O. Meirik, "Steroid Hormone Contraception and Bone Mineral Density: A Cross-Sectional Study in an International Population," *Obstetrics and Gynecology* 95 (2000): 736–744.

Piccinino, L. J., and W. D. Mosher, "Trends in Contraceptive Use in the United States: 1982–1995," *Family Planning Perspectives* 30, no. 1 (1998): 4–10, 46.

Pike, M. C., and R. K. Ross, "Breast Cancer," *British Medical Bulletin* 40, no. 4 (1984): 351–354.

Polderman, K. H., C. D. A. Stehouwer, G. J. van Kamp, C. G. Schalkwijk, and L. J. G. Gooren, "Modulation of Plasma Endothelin Levels by the Menstrual Cycle," *Metabolism* 49, no. 5 (2000): 648–650.

Prentice, R. L., "On the Ability of Blood Pressure Effects to Explain the Relation Between Oral Contraceptives and Cardiovascular Disease," *American Journal of Epidemiology* 127, no. 2 (1988): 213–219.

Price, H., "Deaths from Venous Thromboembolism Associated with Combined Oral Contraceptives," *The Lancet* 350 (August 9, 1997): 450.

Radvany, R. M., N. Vaisrub, C. Ober, K. M. Patel, and F. Hecht, "The Human Sex Ratio: Increase in First-Born Males to Parents with Shared HLA-DR Antigens," *Tissue Antigens* 29, no. 1 (1987): 34–42.

Rako, S., *The Hormone of Desire: The Truth About Sexuality, Menopause, and Testosterone.* New York: Harmony Books, 1996.

Rako, S., *The Hormone of Desire: The Truth About Testosterone, Sexuality, and Menopause.* New York: Three Rivers Press, 1999.

Rako, S., "Testosterone Deficiency: A Key Factor in the Increased Cardiovascular Risk to Women Following Hysterectomy or with Natural Aging?" *Journal of Women's Health* 7 (1998): 825–829.

Rako, S., "Testosterone Supplemental Therapy After Hysterectomy With or Without Concomitant Oophorectomy: Estrogen Alone is Not Enough," *Journal of Women's Health and Gender-Based Medicine* 9, no. 8 (2000): 917–923.

Rako, S., and H. Mazer, *Semrad: The Heart of a Therapist.* New York and London: Jason Aronson Publishers, 1980; reissued Scribner and Aronson, 1983, 1988.

Rees, H. D., R. W. Bonsall, and R. P. Michael, "Pre-optic and Hypothalamic Neurons Accumulate [³H] medroxyprogesterone Acetate in Male Cynomolgus Monkeys," *Life Sciences* 39 (1986): 1353–1359.

Riman, T., P. W. Dickman, S. Nilsson, N. Correia, H. Nordlinder, C. M. Magnusson, E. Weiderpass, and I. P. Persson, "Hormone Replacement Therapy and the Risk of Invasive Epithelial Ovarian Cancer in Swedish Women," *Journal of the National Cancer Institute* 94, no. 7 (2002): 497–504.

Rosendaal, F. R., F. M. Helmerhorst, and J. P. Vandenbroucke, "Female Hormones and Thrombosis," *Arteriosclerosis Thrombosis and Vascular Biology* 22, no. 2 (2002): 201–210.

Ross, R. K., A. Paganini-Hill, P. C. Wan, and M. C. Pike, "Effect of Hormone Replacement Therapy on Breast Cancer Risk: Estrogen Versus Estrogen Plus Progestin," *Journal of the National Cancer Institute* 92, no. 4 (2000): 328–332.

Ross, R. K., and M. C. Pike, "Re: Effect of Hormone Replacement Therapy on Breast Cancer Risk: Estrogen Versus Estrogen Plus Progestin," *Journal of the National Cancer Institute* 92, no. 13 (2000): 1100A–1101A.

Rowan, J., "'Estrophasic' Dosing: A New Concept in Oral Contraceptive Therapy," *American Journal of Obstetrics and Gynecology* 180, no. 2/part 2 (1999): S302–306.

Russell, J. F., G. M. Switz, and K. Thompson, "Olfactory Influences on the Human Menstrual Cycle," *Pharmacology and Biochemical Behavior* 13 (1980): 737–738.

Sangi-Haghpeykar, H., A. N. Poindexter, L. Bateman, and J. R. Ditmore, "Experiences of Injectable Contraceptive Users in an Urban Setting," *Obstetrics and Gynecology* 88 (1996): 227–233.

Santos, C., N. Munoz, S. Klug, M. Almonte, I. Guerrero, M. Alvarez, C. Velarde, O. Galdos, M. Castillo, J. Walboomers, C. Meijer, and E. Caceres, "HPV Types and Cofactors Causing Cervical Cancer in Peru," *British Journal of Cancer* 28, no. 7 (2001): 966–971.

Scanlan, J. M., J. J. Werner, R. L. Legg, and M. L. Laudenslager, "Natural Killer Cell Activity is Reduced in Association with Oral Contraceptive Use," *Psychoneuroendocrinology* 20, no. 3 (1995): 281–287.

Schairer, C., J. Lubin, R. Troisi, S. Sturgeon, L. Brinton, and R. Hoover, "Menopausal Estrogen and Estrogen-Progestin Replacement Therapy and Breast Cancer Risk," *Journal of the American Medical Association* 283, no. 4 (2000): 485–491.

Scharrer, B., "Neurosecretion XIII. The Ultrastructure of the Corpus Cardiacum of the Insect *Leucophaea Maderae*," *Zeitschrift fur Zellforschung* 60 (1963): 761–796.

Scharrer, B., and E. Scharrer, "Neurosecretion VI. A Comparison Between the Intercerebralis-Cardiacum-Allatum System of the Insects and the Hypothalamo-Hypophyseal System of the Vertebrates," *The Biological Bulletin* 87 (December 1944): 242–251.

Schiff, I., "Use of Oral Contraceptives by Women Who Smoke: Introduction," *American Journal of Obstetrics and Gynecology* 180, no. 6/part 2 (1999): S341–S342.

Schmidt, P. J., L. K. Nieman, M. A. Danaceau, L. F. Adams, and D. R. Rubinow, "Differential Behavioral Effects of Gonadal Steroids in Women with and in Those Without Premenstrual Syndrome," *New England Journal of Medicine* 338, no. 4 (1998): 209–216.

Scholes, D., A. Z. Lacroix, S. M. Ott, L. E. Ichikawa, and W. E. Barlow, "Bone Mineral Density in Women Using Depot Medroxyprogesterone Acetate for Contraception," *Obstetrics and Gynecology* 93, no. 2 (1999): 233–238.

Seaman, B., *The Doctors' Case Against the Pill*. Alameda, California: Hunter House, 1994.

Shlipak, M. G., B. G. Angeja, A. S. Go, P. D. Frederick, J. G. Canto, and D. Grady, for the National Registry of Myocardial Infarction-3 Investigators, "Hormone Therapy and In-Hospital Survival After Myocardial Infarction in Postmenopausal Women," *Circulation* 104 (November 6, 2001): 2300–2304.

Silberstein, S. D., "The Role of Sex Hormones in Headache," *Neurology* 42/Supplement 2 (1992): 37–42.

Silberstein, S. D., and G. R. Merriam, "Estrogens, Progestins, and Headache," *Neurology* 41 (1991): 786–793.

Skegg, D. C. G., E. A. Noonan, C. Paul, G. F. Spears, O. Meirik, and D. B. Thomas, "Depot Medroxyprogesterone Acetate and Breast Cancer: A Pooled Analysis of the WHO and New Zealand Studies," *Journal of the American Medical Association* 273, no. 10 (1995): 799–804.

Slone, D., S. Shapiro, D. W. Kaufman, L. Rosenberg, O. S. Miettinen, and P. D. Stolley, "Risk of Myocardial Infarction in Relation to Current and Discontinued Use of Oral Contraceptive," *New England Journal of Medicine* 305 (August 20, 1981): 420–424.

Smith, G. D., and J. Pekkanen, "Should There Be a Moratorium on the Use of Cholesterol Lowering Drugs?" *British Medical Journal* 304 (February 15, 1992): 431–434.

Somerville, B. W., "The Role of Estradiol Withdrawal in the Etiology of Menstrual Migraine," *Neurology* 22 (1972): 355–365.

Speroff, L., R. H. Glass, and N. G. Kase, *Clinical Gynecologic Endocrinology and Infertility.* Baltimore and Philadelphia: Lippincott, Williams & Wilkins, 1999.

Spitzer, W. O., M. A. Lewis, L. A. Heinemann, M. Thorogood, and K. D. MacRae, "Third Generation Oral Contraceptives and Risk of Venous Thromboembolic Disorders: An International Case-control Study," *British Medical Journal* 312 (January 13, 1996): 83–88.

Stadel, B. V., "Oral Contraceptives and Cardiovascular Disease," *New England Journal of Medicine* 305 (September 17, 1981): 672–677.

Stanford, J. L., "Oral Contraceptives and Neoplasia of the Ovary," *Contraception* 43, no. 6 (1991): 543–556.

Stone, N. J., R. I. Levy, D. S. Frederickson, and J. Verter, "Coronary Artery Disease in 116 Kindred with Familial Type II Hyperlipoproteinemia," *Circulation* 49 (1974): 476–488.

Sulak, P. J., "Endometrial Cancer and Hormone Replacement Therapy. Appropriate Use of Progestins to Oppose Endogenous and

Exogenous Estrogen," *Endocrinology and Metabolism Clinics of North America* 26, no. 2 (1997): 399–412.

Sullivan, J. L., "Coronary Artery Disease in Men and Women," *New England Journal of Medicine* 305, no. 25 (1981): 1531.

Sullivan, J. L., "Iron and the Sex Difference in Heart Disease Risk," *The Lancet* (June 13, 1981): 1293–1294.

Sullivan, J. L., "The Iron Paradigm of Ischemic Heart Disease," *American Heart Journal* 117, no. 5 (1989): 1177–1188.

Sullivan, J. L., "Iron Versus Cholesterol—Perspectives on the Iron and Heart Disease Debate," *Journal of Clinical Epidemiology* 49, no. 12 (1996): 1345–1352.

Tanis, B. C., M. A. A. J. van den Bosch, J. M. Kemmeren, V. M. Cats, F. M. Helmerhorst, A. Algra, Y. van der Graaf, and F. R. Rosendaal, "Oral Contraceptives and the Risk of Myocardial Infarction," *New England Journal of Medicine* 345, no. 25 (2001): 1787–1793.

Templeman, C., H. Boyd, and S. P. Hertweck, "Depotmedroxy-progesterone Acetate Use and Weight Gain Among Adolescents," *Journal of Pediatric and Adolescent Gynecology* 13 (2000): 45–46.

Thomas, S. L., and C. Ellertson, "Nuisance or Natural and Healthy: Should Monthly Menstruation be Optional for Women?" *The Lancet* 355 (March 11, 2000): 922–924.

Tomer, A., A. D. Schreiber, R. McMillan, D. B. Cines, S. A. Burstein, A. Thiessen, and L. A. Harker, "Menstrual Cyclic Thrombocytopenia," *British Journal of Haematology* 71 (1989): 519–524.

Tuomainen, T-P., K. Punnonen, K. Nyyssönen, and J. T. Salonen, "Association Between Body Iron Stores and the Risk of Acute Myocardial Infarction in Men," *Circulation* 97 (1998): 1461–1466.

Tuomainen, T-P., R. Salonen, K. Nyyssönen, and J. T. Salonen, "Cohort Study of Relation Between Donating Blood and Risk of Myocardial Infarction in 2682 Men in Eastern Finland," *British Medical Journal* 314 (March 15, 1997): 793–794.

Ursin, G., C. Li, and M. C. Pike, "Should Women with a Family History of Breast Cancer Avoid Use of Oral Contraceptives?" *Epidemiology* 11, no. 5 (2000): 615–616.

USDA Nutrient Data Base for Standard Reference, Release 12, 1998.

Vandenbrouke, J. P., K. W. Bloemenkamp, F. R. Rosendall, and F. M. Helmerhorst, "Incidence of Venous Thromboembolism in Users of Combined Oral Contraception. Risk Is Particularly High with First Use of Oral Contraceptives," *British Medical Journal* 320 (January 1, 2000): 57–58.

Vessey, M. P., M. Lawless, K. McPherson, and D. Yeates, "Neoplasia of the Cervix Uteri and Contraception: A Possible Adverse Effect of the Pill," *The Lancet* (October 22, 1983): 930–934.

Warner, P., and J. Bancroft, "Mood, Sexuality, Oral Contraceptives and the Menstrual Cycle," *Journal of Psychosomatic Research* 32, nos. 4/5 (1988): 417–427.

Wedekind, C., and S. Furi, "Body Odour Preferences in Men and Women: Do They Aim for Specific MHC Combinations or Simply Heterozygosity?" *Proceedings of the Royal Society of London* 264 (1997): 1471–1479.

Wedekind, C., T. Seebeck, F. Bettens, and J. Paepke, "MHC-dependent Mate Preferences in Humans," *Proceedings of the Royal Society of London* 260 (1995): 245–249.

Weiss, N., "Third-generation Oral Contraceptives: How Risky?" *The Lancet* 346 (December 15, 1995): 1570.

Weisz, J., G. T. Ross, and P. D. Stolley, "Report of the Public Board of Inquiry on Depo-Provera (Rockville, Maryland)," United States Food and Drug Administration, 1984.

Whiting, S. J., and B. Lemke, "Excess Retinol Intake May Explain the High Incidence of Osteoporosis in Northern Europe," *Nutrition Reviews* 57, no. 6 (1999): 192–195.

Whittemore, A. S., R. Harris, and J. Itnyre, "Characteristics Relating to Ovarian Cancer Risk: Collaborative Analysis of 12 US Case-control

Studies. II. Invasive Epithelial Ovarian Cancers in White Women," *American Journal of Epidemiology* 36, no. 10 (1992): 1184–1203.

WHO Collaborative Study of Neoplasia and Steroid Contraceptives, "Depot-medroxyprogesterone Acetate (DMPA) and Risk of Endo-metrial Cancer," *International Journal of Cancer* 49 (1991): 186.

WHO Collaborative Study of Neoplasia and Steroid Contraceptives, "Depot-Medroxyprogesterone Acetate (DMPA) and Risk of Epithelial Ovarian Cancer," *International Journal of Cancer* 49 (1991): 191–195.

WHO Collaborative Study of Neoplasia and Steroid Contraceptives, "Depot-Medroxyprogesterone Acetate (DMPA) and Risk of Invasive Squamous Cell Cervical Cancer," *Contraception* 45 (1992): 299–312.

World Health Organization, "A Multicentre Comparative Study of Serum Lipids and Apolipoproteins in Long-Term Users of DMPA and a Control Group of IUD Users," *Contraception* 47 (1993): 177–191.

Wiest, W. G., M. O. Pulkkinen, J. Sauvage, and A. I. Csapo, "Plasma Progesterone Levels During Saline-induced Abortion," *Journal of Clinical Endocrinology and Metabolism* 30 (1970): 774–777.

World Health Organization Collaborative Study of Cardiovascular Disease and Steroid Hormone Contraception, "Effect of Different Progestagens in Low Oestrogen Oral Contraceptives on Venous Thromboembolic Disease," *The Lancet* 346 (December 16, 1995): 1582–1588.

World Health Organization: WHO Collaborative Study of Neoplasia and Steroid Contraceptives, "Invasive Cervical Cancer and Combined Oral Contraceptives," *British Medical Journal* 290 (March 30, 1985): 961–965.

Writing Group for the PEPI, "Effects of Estrogen or Estrogen/ Progestin Regimens on Heart Disease Risk Factors in Postmenopausal Women. The Postmenopausal Estrogen/Progestin Interventions (PEPI) Trial," *Journal of the American Medical Association* 273 (1995): 199–208.

Writing Group for the PEPI, "Effects of Estrogen or Estrogen/ Progestin Regimens on Endometrial Histology in Postmenopausal

Women. The Postmenopausal Estrogen/Progestin Interventions (PEPI) Trial," *Journal of the American Medical Association* 275 (1996): 370–375.

Writing Group for the Women's Health Initiative Investigators, "Risks and Benefits of Estrogen Plus Progestin in Healthy Postmenopausal Women," *Journal of the American Medical Association* 288 (July 17, 2002): 321–333.

Wyatt, K., P. Dimmock, P. Jones, M. Obhrai, and S. O'Brien, "Efficacy of Progesterone and Progestogens in Management of Premenstrual Syndrome: Systematic Review," *British Medical Journal* 323 (October 6, 2001): 776–780.

Yen, S. S. C., and R. B. Jaffe, eds., *Reproductive Endocrinology*. Philadelphia: W.B. Saunders Company, 1991.

Zimmerman, A. W., "Hormones and Epilepsy," *Neurologic Clinics* 4, no. 4 (1986): 853–861.

Index

About the Author

SUSAN RAKO, M.D., is the author of the ground-breaking book *The Hormone of Desire: The Truth About Testosterone, Sexuality, and Menopause,* which rocketed her to international prominence as a preeminent authority on testosterone deficiency and supplementation for women. An expert in the field of women's hormonal health and a devout defender of women's health rights, Dr. Rako is a Boston-based psychiatrist who has been in private practice for thirty years. After graduation from Albert Einstein College of Medicine, she trained and taught at Harvard Medical School's Massachusetts Mental Health Center.

Dr. Rako is at work on a collection of essays and stories from her life. Visit her website at http://www.susanrako.com.